T0297936

Updates in Surgery

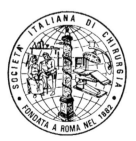

Gilberto Poggioli
Editor

Ulcerative Colitis

Foreword by
Marco Montorsi

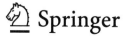

Editor
Gilberto Poggioli
Department of Medical and Surgical Sciences
University of Bologna
General Surgery Unit, Department of Digestive Diseases
S. Orsola-Malpighi Hospital
Bologna, Italy

The publication and the distribution of this volume have been supported by the Italian Society of Surgery

ISSN 2280-9848   ISSN 2281-0854 (electronic)
Updates in Surgery
ISBN 978-88-470-3976-6   ISBN 978-88-470-3977-3 (eBook)

DOI 10.1007/978-88-470-3977-3

Library of Congress Control Number: 2018948376

Cover design: eStudio Calamar S.L.
External publishing product development: Scienzaperta, Novate Milanese (Milan), Italy
Typesetting: Graphostudio, Milan, Italy

This Springer imprint is published by Springer Nature
The registered company is Springer-Verlag Italia S.r.l.
The registered company address is Via Decembrio 28, I-20137 Milan

Foreword

The spirit of the Italian Society of Surgery's Biennial Reports, established almost 25 years ago and one of its most important editorial activities, has always been to deal with highly relevant topics characterized by important diagnostic and therapeutic developments, assigned to recognized experts representing consolidated national surgical schools.

This is also the case of the present monograph on ulcerative colitis, addressed for the first time in this series: the Society's Executive Board has decided to assign the topic to Prof. Gilberto Poggioli in representation of the glorious School of Bologna.

After the 2009 monograph on the treatment of Crohn's Disease by Prof. Roberto Tersigni, the other major chapter of inflammatory bowel diseases – namely, ulcerative colitis – is now presented.

With the qualified contribution of colleagues from the University of Bologna and the S. Orsola-Malpighi Hospital, Prof. Poggioli has divided this complex area into clear and well-structured chapters that will help readers find their way and locate effective answers to the numerous clinical questions that this disease still poses today.

Great space has also been devoted to the more exquisitely surgical aspects of both technique and indication, without neglecting the great emerging field of minimally invasive methods.

Although the current trend is to progressively concentrate the management of this condition in referral centers offering all areas of expertise and able to maintain high volumes of activity, I am sure that all Italian surgeons will find great interest and frequent consultation of this work on which I congratulate all the authors on behalf of the whole Society.

Milan, September 2018   Marco Montorsi
                                    President, Italian Society of Surgery

v

Preface

The biennial report on ulcerative colitis which the Italian Society of Surgery (SIC) entrusted to me represents an honor as well as a tribute to the surgeons of the University of Bologna.

Exactly sixty years later, a chief of surgery at the University of Bologna is invited to speak on ulcerative colitis at the SIC congress. In fact, it was Gaetano Placitelli who first spoke about the systematic treatment of this disease at the SIC Congress in Genoa in 1958. Two years later, his fellows, Leonardo Possati and Antonello Franchini, published an awesome text (*La colite ulcerosa*, Bologna, 1960) which, for the first time in Italy, exhaustively discussed the disease from the etiopathogenetic as well as from the clinical, surgical and anatomopathological points of view.

Many years have passed since 1958; however, the school that Gaetano Placitelli founded has always considered inflammatory bowel diseases to be a scientific, didactic and patient-oriented topic. Knowledge regarding this topic has grown and experience has increased but, ever since 1958, Bologna has created what today we tend to call multidisciplinary teams. Under the direction of Professors Giuseppe Labò and Luigi Barbara and then Giorgio Assuero Lanfranchi, an osmosis between medical and surgical groups originated which has brought many scientific milestones to Bologna. The structural turning point arrived, however, with Prof. Massimo Campieri who, after having spent a long period of time in Oxford under the mythical Sydney Truelove, brought to Bologna this method, not only of working, but of reasoning in a joint teamwise fashion. Then, in 1981, my Maestro, Giuseppe Gozzetti who, together with Luigi Barbara and Massimo Campieri, put together a group of which I was a part directly from the beginning. Already in the 1980s, this group was characterized by the impressive number (first in Italy) of operations carried out for ulcerative colitis, in particular the ileoanal-pouch anastomosis, only a few years after the technique had been proposed in London at St. Mark's Hospital by Sir Alan Parks and John Nicholls.

All this, together with internships at the Cleveland Clinic and the Lahey Clinic, led to close friendships and international collaboration which, in turn, led to the first congress "New Trends in Pelvic Pouch Procedures" held in Bologna in 1989 in collaboration with the Cleveland and Mayo Clinics. It was the first occasion, not only for evaluating surgical techniques and complications, possible technical variants and future problems which the new type of surgery could involve, but, for the first time, to discuss the pathophysiology of ileoanal anastomosis, evaluating not only the anatomical changes, but also the quality of life as well as the physiological, morphological and functional modifications which derive from the surgery.

The rest is recent history and keeps up with the experiences of the largest world centers which are expert in this sector, bringing many of us to act as tutors in other Italian centers and to be a part of the drawing up of new guidelines of many scientific societies regarding the medical and surgical therapy for ulcerative colitis.

Therefore, I take the occasion of presenting this book as a tribute to Bologna, to its Alma Mater Studiorum University, to its most important hospital, Policlinico S. Orsola-Malpighi, and to the colleagues who, in the past forty years, have dedicated their energy, passion and competence to improving and increasingly understanding the behavior, varieties, diagnosis and therapy of ulcerative colitis, a disease which is on the increase in the Western world.

Bologna, September 2018   Gilberto Poggioli

Contents

All web addresses have been checked and were correct at time of printing.

Contributors

Luca Boschi General Surgery Unit, Department of Digestive Diseases, S. Orsola-Malpighi Hospital, Bologna, Italy

Carlo Calabrese Department of Medical and Surgical Sciences, University of Bologna, S. Orsola-Malpighi Hospital, Bologna, Italy

Andrea Calafiore Department of Medical and Surgical Sciences, University of Bologna, S. Orsola-Malpighi Hospital, Bologna, Italy

Lucia Calandrini Department of Medical and Surgical Sciences, University of Bologna, S. Orsola-Malpighi Hospital, Bologna, Italy

Massimo Campieri Department of Medical and Surgical Sciences, University of Bologna, S. Orsola-Malpighi Hospital, Bologna, Italy

Alberta Cappelli Radiology Unit, Department of Diagnostic and Preventive Medicine, S. Orsola-Malpighi Hospital, Bologna, Italy

Maurizio Coscia General Surgery Unit, Department of Digestive Diseases, S. Orsola-Malpighi Hospital, Bologna, Italy

Antonietta D'Errico Department of Experimental Diagnostic and Specialty Medicine, University of Bologna, S. Orsola-Malpighi Hospital, Bologna, Italy

Massimo P. Di Simone Department of Medical and Surgical Sciences, University of Bologna, S. Orsola-Malpighi Hospital, Bologna, Italy

Lorenzo Gentilini General Surgery Unit, Department of Digestive Diseases, S. Orsola-Malpighi Hospital, Bologna, Italy

Federico Ghignone General Surgery Unit, Department of Digestive Diseases, S. Orsola-Malpighi Hospital, Bologna, Italy

Paolo Gionchetti Department of Medical and Surgical Sciences, University of Bologna, S. Orsola-Malpighi Hospital, Bologna, Italy

Silvio Laureti Department of Medical and Surgical Sciences,
University of Bologna, S. Orsola-Malpighi Hospital, Bologna, Italy

Deborah Malvi Pathology Unit, Department of Diagnostic and Preventive
Medicine, S. Orsola-Malpighi Hospital, Bologna, Italy

Marta Mazza Department of Medical and Surgical Sciences,
University of Bologna, S. Orsola-Malpighi Hospital, Bologna, Italy

Gilberto Poggioli Department of Medical and Surgical Sciences,
University of Bologna, S. Orsola-Malpighi Hospital, Bologna, Italy

Chiara Praticò Interventional Ultrasound Unit, Department of Organ Failure
and Transplantation, S. Orsola-Malpighi Hospital, Bologna, Italy

Hana Privitera Hrustemovic Department of Medical and Surgical Sciences,
University of Bologna, S. Orsola-Malpighi Hospital, Bologna, Italy

Nicola Renzi Department of Medical and Surgical Sciences,
University of Bologna, S. Orsola-Malpighi Hospital, Bologna, Italy

Fernando Rizzello Department of Medical and Surgical Sciences,
University of Bologna, S. Orsola-Malpighi Hospital, Bologna, Italy

Matteo Rottoli Department of Medical and Surgical Sciences,
University of Bologna, S. Orsola-Malpighi Hospital, Bologna, Italy

Marco Salice Department of Medical and Surgical Sciences,
University of Bologna, S. Orsola-Malpighi Hospital, Bologna, Italy

Carla Serra Interventional Ultrasound Unit, Department of Organ Failure
and Transplantation, S. Orsola-Malpighi Hospital, Bologna, Italy

Federica Ugolini General Surgery Unit, Department of Digestive Diseases,
S. Orsola-Malpighi Hospital, Bologna, Italy

Laura Vittori General Surgery Unit, Department of Digestive Diseases,
S. Orsola-Malpighi Hospital, Bologna, Italy

History of Ulcerative Colitis

1

Gilberto Poggioli, Marco Salice, Nicola Renzi,
and Massimo Campieri

1.1   Introduction

Ulcerative colitis (UC) is an idiopathic inflammatory disease limited to the
colon [1] that extends proximally from the rectum. It is a chronic condition
which presents primarily in the third and fourth decades of life [2] with bloody
diarrhea, rectal urgency and abdominal pain [3].

The incidence and prevalence of UC, along with Crohn's disease, is highest
in westernized nations, such as Canada, Northern Europe and Australia. In
recent years, a rise in the incidence and prevalence was observed in developing
nations, probably related to a change in environmental risk factors, such as diet,
microbial exposure, sanitation, lifestyle behavior, medications and pollution
exposure [4].

Despite years of investigation, the roots of UC have yet to be identified.
The strongest modifying factors known so far include: cigarette smoking [5];
appendectomy, which seems to have a protective effect [6]; family history of
inflammatory bowel disease (IBD), which is the greatest risk factor for the
development of UC and Crohn's disease [7].

1.2   Ancient Times

The earliest descriptions of chronic diarrhea date back to ancient Chinese
medicine. In 722 BCE the yellow emperor's Canon of internal medicine described

N. Renzi (✉)
Department of Medical and Surgical Sciences, University of Bologna, S. Orsola-Malpighi
Hospital
Bologna, Italy
e-mail: nicola.renzi4@unibo.it

G. Poggioli (Ed), *Ulcerative Colitis,*
Updates in Surgery
DOI: 10.1007/978-88-470-3977-3_1, © Springer-Verlag Italia 2019

symptoms (abdominal pain, diarrhea, rectal bleeding) of a disease resembling UC [8]. In the 4th century BCE, the great Greek physician Hippocrates of Kos gave a description of a bloody, mucus-streaked stool [9] and, in the first century CE, Aretaeus of Cappadocia [10] noted a distinct type of "foul evacuation", occurring more often in women than in men. Even if both physicians recognized different forms of diarrhea, they could not differentiate between infectious and non-infectious causes.

1.3   Discovery

1.3.1   First Case Reports

It has been suggested that, in 1745, Prince Charles, the Young Pretender to the throne of Great Britain, suffered from UC and cured himself by adopting a milk-free diet [11].

In the 17th century the English physician Thomas Sydenham gave a detailed description of cases of "bloody flux", a condition characterized by the presence of blood mixed with loose, watery stools. This illness was probably of infectious origin, although it is impossible to verify whether instances of UC were included [12].

In the 18th century, another English physician, Burch, reported the case of a 40-year-old man who developed persistent "bloody flux" in 1756 and also experienced bouts of jaundice, fever and episodic abdominal pain 5 years later. In the following years he also experienced sore eyes and joint pain suggesting extra-intestinal manifestations. The symptoms continued intermittently until the patient died in 1774. The case report suggested the possibility of non-specific inflammatory bowel disease complicated by primary sclerosing cholangitis [13].

In 1793, in his *The Morbid Anatomy of Some of the Most Important Parts of the Human Body*, the pathologist Matthew Baillie (1761–1823) suggested that, according to his autopsy descriptions, people were dying from UC in the latter part of the 18th century [14].

In 1859, Samuel Wilks (1824–1911) of London was the first physician to use the term "ulcerative colitis" in a case report. The patient was a 42-year-old woman who presented with diarrhea and fever, which was initially diagnosed as arsenic poisoning. The autopsy showed transmural ulcerative inflammation of the entire colon and terminal ileum, initially designated as simple ulcerative colitis, but which was later revealed to be a case of Crohn's disease [15].

The 1875 case report of Wilks and Moxon, regarding a young woman who had died from severe bloody diarrhea and whose autopsy showed ulceration and inflammation of the colonic mucosa, was probably the first instance of UC [16].

Around the same period of time, similar reports circulated in Europe such as the description by William Henry Allchin (1846–1912) of London in 1885 of the extensive denudation of the colon in a young woman who died after 6 weeks of diarrhea [17] and a series of cases of "ulcerative colitis" published by Sir William Hale White of London (1857–1949). It is from this report that the term "ulcerative colitis" entered into the general medical vocabulary.

1.3.2   First Therapeutic and Diagnostic Attempts

Surgical management of UC began to emerge around the last decade of the nineteenth century.

In 1893, the English surgeon Arthur William Mayo Robson (1853–1933), Professor of Surgery at Yorkshire College of Victoria University attempted to treat the inflamed bowel of a 37-year-old female patient with bloody diarrhea by means of a temporary inguinal colostomy permitting daily irrigations with ipecacuanha and tincture of *Hamamelis* and, later, with a boracic acid solution, allowing the closure of the colostomy. This was performed using a left inguinal incision of the abdominal wall through which the sigmoidal colon was fixed and opened externally [18].

In 1902, Robert Fulton Weir (1838–1927) of New York was the first to perform an appendicostomy in a patient with UC to allow colonic irrigation with antimicrobial solutions (5% solution of methylene blue alternating with a 5% solution of silver nitrate or bismuth). Even if it did not achieve complete functional exclusion of the colon, Weir's appendicostomy remained the standard of care in severe colitis for years [19].

In 1907, John Percy Lockhart-Mummery (1875–1957) reported cases of carcinoma of the colon in 7 of 36 patients in his series of surgical cases of UC. In the same paper, he was the first doctor to demonstrate that the recently developed illuminated proctosigmoidoscope was a safe and invaluable tool for colonic mucosa evaluation and diagnosis.

1.3.3   1909 London Symposium

In 1909 the Royal Society of Medicine in London held a symposium where over 300 cases of patients admitted to London hospitals (Guy's, London St Bartholomew's, St George, St Thomas, St Mary and Westminster) from 1883 and 1908, with severe inflammation of the colon, were presented and discussed. The conference shed some light on different aspects of the disease, such as risk factors (early adult and middle age), common presenting symptoms (diarrhea and hemorrhage), complications (141 patients had died from perforation of the colon, hemorrhage, liver disease, septic infection, pulmonary embolism and malnutrition) and therapeutic attempts. Medical treatment included a great variety of options, such as "slop diets", Sydenham's remedy (3 pints daily of milk soured by lactic acid), astringents, opium, tincture of *Hamamelis*, rectal instillations of boracic acid, silver nitrate or creolin administered to control a presumed infection.

The most popular operation at the time was appendicostomy or, if the appendix had been removed, a valvular cecostomy followed by colonic irrigations. Etiologic speculations focused mainly on bacteriological possibilities [20]. In March of the same year, the British Medical Journal published the Herbert P. Hawkins "Address on the natural history of ulcerative colitis and its bearing on treatment". This lecture read before the Bristol Medico-Chirurgical Society explained that "nothing can be done until the natural history of the disease is understood". He indicated that the active bacterial agents responsible for the disease should be found so that they could be controlled [21].

1.4   1910s–1950s

1.4.1   Breakthroughs and Growing Interest

In the decades following 1909, reports of cases of UC started coming in from all over the world and in 1913 at the Paris Congress of Medicine, the disease was one of the principal subjects discussed. In the same year, the first radiological appearance of UC was described independently by Sterlin and Kienbock, and the first American case report was published by Bassler of New York [22].

By the 1930s, the first descriptions of pediatric UC started to emerge, such as the 1923 Helmholz of Mayo Clinic report of the clinical features of the disease in five children aged 8 to 15 [23] and the 1940 Mayo Clinic report of a total of 95 children with UC [24].

The impact of UC on growth and sexual development in children was also recognized; in 1939, Davidson of the Bronx Memorial Hospital reported impaired growth in children affected by the disease and, in 1937, Welch et al. tried to explain nutritional deficiencies by demonstrating substantial fecal losses of proteins and electrolytes [25].

Several breakthroughs were made, such as the first demonstrations of familial predisposition to UC by Spriggs in 1934 and Moltke in 1937, who recorded five families with multiple instances of the disease (mother/daughter in two families; brother/sister in two families and father/daughter in one family) [26].

In 1915, another important milestone was reached with Hewitt's association between chronic UC and polyps [27] and, subsequently, in 1948 when Wengensteen recognized that UC heralded colon cancer [28].

1.4.2   Medical Therapy

Medical interventions included several experimental treatments such as "organotherapy", which consisted of feeding raw porcine small bowel to patients in the hope of replacing a lack of a hypothetical factor [29]. Another treatment proposed was "ionization therapy", which involved irrigating the bowel with a zinc solution and then running an electric current through the solution [30]. Furthermore, in 1923, in his paper on UC, Strauss from Berlin suggested that a bland diet and blood transfusion could be helpful [31]. Psychogenic factors were formally implicated in UC in the reports of Murray and Sullivan who had been impressed with a chronological relationship between emotional disturbances and the onset of bowel symptoms in men and women with significant emotional disturbances involving their marriage, home life and interpersonal relationships. Psychiatric precepts during the 1930s and 1940s emphasized an UC personality described as "immaturity of the patient, indecisiveness, over-dependence and inhibited interpersonal relationships together with critical emotional events including the loss of a loved one, feeling of social rejection and maternal dominance".

Psychotherapy was an important part of medical treatment during the 1930s–1950s. Grace, Pinsky, and Wolff reported lower operability rates, fewer serious complications, and lower mortality rates in 34 patients with UC treated by stress control therapy. However, in a series of 70 patients with severe UC treated by psychoanalytically oriented psychotherapy for three months, no specific value was observed in preventing surgical intervention on severe recurrences. Years later, Feldman et al. found no evidence of a psychogenic causation in a controlled study of 34 patients with UC [32].

1.4.3   Surgical Treatment

Initially, surgical treatment of UC was sporadic and mostly experimental; however, after 1930, surgical interventions gradually became standardized. Several of these techniques were later abandoned, but a few are still in use today.

Some of these abandoned experimental surgical treatments included Neumann's description of pneumoperitoneum and Dennis's vagotomy as simple and effective therapeutic procedures in apparently intractable cases of chronic UC. In 1943, Neumann described seven cases of UC treated with therapeutic pneumoperitoneum. The technique consisted of inserting a needle into the left iliac fossa, at one inch from the umbilicus, and inserting oxygen or air at a pressure of 2–3 cm water with the same apparatus already in use for pneumothorax; the procedure was repeated once or twice weekly for months until the patient had sufficient clinical relief [33]. In 1947, Dennis et al. reported the results obtained by a vagotomy performed on patients with UC. The technique consisted of dividing the vagal nerves by means of a seventh intercostal anterior space incision; the patients were followed up for months [34].

Surgical interventions which have withstood the test of time include ileostomy, and subtotal or total colectomy.

1.4.3.1 Ileostomy

The first surgeon suggesting ileostomy to treat UC was John Young Brown (1865–1919) who, in 1913, suggested that placing the large bowel on complete physiological rest was necessary for the treatment of the inflammatory bowel disease. Brown's procedure, in adjunct to cecostomy for bowel irrigation obtained after appendix removal, consisted of a complete division of the ileum near the ileocecal valve and a flush terminal ileostomy, protruding some centimeters and fixed in a mid-line laparotomy. The intestinal contents were kept away from the skin of the abdominal wall by a catheter sewn in place. After the patient had recovered sufficiently, the catheter was removed and the ileostomy "matured" as a result of serositis secondary to the caustic ileal contents [35].

Subsequently, many surgeons, including Brown, started to divert only the fecal stream with an ileostomy, without a stoma for irrigation purposes. This procedure also had the advantage of being reversible, by closing the stoma. It was also noted that, even after a prolonged large bowel rest, closing the ileostomy was often followed by a flare-up of the colitis.

Ileostomy according to Brown provided total fecal diversion, but presented a high rate of complications, such as dehydration, hydroelectrolytic disorders and skin excoriation in the short term, and mechanical problems in the long term (retraction, stenosis, prolapse, parastomal hernia). Furthermore, since this operation was undertaken with reluctance and was reserved for critically ill patients, it was associated with high mortality [36].

The use of ileostomy spread after the introduction of easier to manage devices and after the development of an alternative technique for fashioning the ileostomy as proposed by Sir Bryan Brooke in London.

Bryan Nicholas Brooke (1915–1998) Professor of Surgery at Queen Elizabeth Hospital in Birmingham described a new technique for everting ileostomy in order to minimize skin excoriation; it was adopted worldwide and continues to be used today. The procedure consisted of a partial intussusception of the external part of the ileal segment of the stoma, allowing protection of the serosa, and reducing stenosis and excessive output. It also facilitated the application of a closely approximated device to the base of the stoma, thereby minimizing the ingress of fluid which could subsequently lead to leakage under the free edge of the stoma device [37]. Furthermore, in the late 1950s the birth and growth of stoma care was pioneered at the Cleveland Clinic in Ohio where the "R.B. Turnbull Wound Ostomy Continence (WOC) School" was born [38].

1.4.3.2 Ileorectal Anastomosis

Total colectomy with ileo-sigmoidal anastomosis for UC was first described in 1903 by Howard Lilienthal (1861–1946) [39] from New York who was, for the most part, known for his interest in thoracic surgery. In 1943, Sir Hugh Berchmans Devine (1878–1959) reported a multiple-stage procedure of partial colectomy and ileo-rectal anastomosis for patients in very poor condition [40]. Doctor Alfred A. Strauss (1881–1971) was an early advocate of the total proctocolectomy and end ileostomy as a definitive treatment for UC. After Strauss presented his results regarding this approach in 1944, it was clear that a multiple-stage procedure consisting of removing the entire colon and rectum was effective and safe in the management of UC. At the same time, the surgeon described the "Koenig Bag" a rubber device which could be bound and sealed to the skin and supported with an elastic belt, designed to prevent bowel contents from reaching the skin around the stoma. This device was named after Mr. Koenig, who had had an ileostomy for UC and helped develop the stoma bag for his own use [41].

In 1948, Richard Cattell (1900–1964) described a three-stage surgical approach: ileostomy, subtotal colectomy and, finally, an abdominoperineal resection of the rectum. In 1949 Miller recommended a two-stage ileostomy and proctocolectomy and, in 1951, Mark M. Ravitch (1910–1989), a leading pediatric surgeon and a pioneer in the United States in the use of mechanical stapling devices for surgery, accomplished the procedure in one stage. Furthermore, Ravitch was an innovator, introducing mucosectomy to the restorative surgical technique (sphincter saving in ileo-anal anastomosis) for managing UC. In 1951, Campbell Gardner (1908–1963) and Gavin Miller (1893–1964) presented a series of 69 patients, who had undergone a one-stage colectomy, consisting of ileostomy and colectomy at the same time. Due to the severity of illness of the study population, mortality occurred in 15% of cases [42].

Total colectomy with ileorectal anastomosis performed for the most part by Devine in Australia [43] and in a more systematic way in the 1950s by Stanley Osborn Aylett (1911–2003) in England did not require ileostomy, restoring intestinal continuity with ileorectal anastomosis. Aylett reported an operative mortality of 5%, and 90% of the patients were restored to health [44].

By contrast, because of the poor results in many patients, the need for additional surgery and the risk of cancer, many surgeons remained skeptical and reluctant to carry out the procedure [45].

1.5   1960s–1990s

1.5.1   Medical Therapy Milestones (Table 1.1)

1.5.1.1 Aminosalicylates

Sulfasalazine (SASP) was first synthesized by Nanna Svartz, a Swedish Professor of Medicine at the Karolinska Institute in Stockholm. It contains sulfapyridine (SP), an antibiotic, and 5-aminosalicyclin acid (5-ASA), an anti-inflammatory, linked by a diazo bond. Dr. Svartz initially used sulfasalazine to treat patients with rheumatoid arthritis, but the results were not encouraging. Unexpectedly when used in patients with UC it led to significant improvement in their diarrhea [46]. She published her first case report in 1942, followed by a large uncontrolled study in 1948, which showed that the majority of patients (70–80%) with mild–moderate UC responded well, but relapse was the rule at drug discontinuation [47]. The efficacy of sulfasalazine was confirmed by Baron in 1962 in the first double blind randomized control trial (RCT) [48] and SASP therefore became the drug of choice for UC all over the world. In 1977, Azad Khan and Sidney Truelove (1913–2002) recognized that the active therapeutic part of SASP was 5-ASA and that the SP functioned as a mere carrier and was also responsible for the majority of the side effects [49].

Another important turning point in the medical therapy of UC was realized by Massimo Campieri of the University of Bologna who demonstrated the superiority of rectally administered 5-ASA to placebo, rectally administered

Table 1.1 Timeline of major historical events in the medical treatment of ulcerative colitis

Year	Author	Active compound
1948	Svartz	Oral sulfasalazine
1955	Truelove	Oral corticosteroids
1962	Lennard-Jones	Topical corticosteroids
1962	Bean	6-MP
1974	Truelove	Azathioprine
1977	Azad Khan	Oral 5-ASA
1981	Campieri	Topical 5-ASA
1994	Lichtiger	Ciclosporin
2005	FDA approved	Infliximab
2012	FDA approved	Adalimumab
2013	FDA approved	Golimumab
2014	FDA approved	Vedolizumab

steroids and oral 5-ASA for the induction of symptomatic, endoscopic and histological improvement and remission [50]. Seventy years after Nanna Svartz's discovery of SASP, salicylates continue to play a central role in the treatment of UC. The few side effects, the relatively low cost and effectiveness make these drugs still competitive even in the era of biological agents. The new oral formulations, by improving patient compliance and allowing treatment of left-sided colitis, may open new horizons for an old drug [51].

1.5.1.2 Corticosteroids

In 1954, Palmer and Kirsner published their experience with corticosteroid use in 120 patients with UC, demonstrating that corticosteroids were able to induce a very rapid symptomatic response but, on the other hand, the authors were unable to induce permanent healing. Of their 120 patients, 35 went into remission (defined as complete resolution of symptoms) and another 57 patients improved. In addition to the clinical effects, the common side effects of corticosteroids were reported (acne, hirsutism, Cushing deformities, hyperglycemia, hypertension and an increased incidence of common and opportunistic infections, the latter being the cause of one death from overwhelming sepsis) [52].

In 1955, Sidney Truelove published the first blinded, controlled trial in UC patients in the British Medical Journal demonstrating improvement and decreased mortality for patients taking corticosteroids when compared to the control subjects. Notably, this very first trial already included some type of rudimentary serial sigmoidoscopic assessments (defined as "normal", "improved" or "no change or worse") in their outcome measures [53].

In 1962, Professor John Lennard-Jones and Sir Francis Avery Jones (St Mark's Hospital, London) published the results of the first double-blind placebo-controlled trial of topical steroids in UC (proctitis). They used both symptomatic and sigmoidoscopic assessment to evaluate outcome and found significant improvement in the patients given steroids topically compared with placebo [54].

A turning point in the management of UC was the 1974 Truelove and Jewell definition of a 5-day intensive intravenous regimen for the treatment of severe attacks of UC. This regimen gave a higher remission-rate than that previously recorded, and failure to respond provided a simple and straightforward indication for surgery without further delay. Finally, early surgery and strict collaboration between the gastroenterologist and the surgeon dramatically reduced mortality [55]. Corticosteroid therapy in new intravenous, oral and topical formulations is still currently in use nowadays.

1.5.1.3 Thiopurines and Ciclosporin

In the 1960s, Bean et al. discovered that mercaptopurine (6-MP) was efficacious in patients with UC [56] and, in the 1970s, azathioprine, another drug of the thiopurine family, was also shown to be effective for treating UC [57]. An unfortunate disadvantage of this particular family of drugs is the risk of complications from bone marrow suppression. In the 1980s it was found that patients with the enzyme methyltransferase (TPMT) were especially at risk for such complications due to decreased drug inactivation. Thus, TPMT gene variation is increasingly being measured in patients before starting azathioprine or 6-MP.

In 1994, intravenous ciclosporin was introduced as the first rescue therapy in patients with severe corticosteroid-resistant UC [58].

1.5.2 Surgical Milestones (Table 1.2)

1.5.2.1 Continent Ileostomy of Kock
A continent ileostomy (known as the Kock pouch) was proposed by Nils Kock in 1969 as an alternative to conventional end ileostomy in order to improve the quality of life of people in whom, despite the great improvements achieved with everted Brooke's ileostomy, physical and psychological difficulties were still common. It consisted of an internal ileal reservoir which stores stools and gas, a stoma outflow and outflow tract needed to intubate and evacuate the content of the reservoir, and a biologic valve interposed between the other two components to act as a pressure barrier to maintain continence. The long-term complications of Kock's pouch were mainly related to the valve mechanism: sliding of the nipple valve, fistula, partial or total prolapse of the valve, necrosis of the valve or the outlet, stricture of the stoma and inflammatory changes in the reservoir

Table 1.2 Timeline of major historical events in the surgical treatment of ulcerative colitis

Year	Author	Surgical procedure
1913	Brown	Ileostomy
1943	Neumann	Pneumoperitoneum
1944	Strauss	Total proctocolectomy and end ileostomy and Koenig Bag
1947	Dennis	Vagotomy
1951	Ravitch	One stage ileorectal anastomosis and ileostomy and mucosectomy
1952	Brooke	Brooke's ileostomy
1953	Turnbull	Stoma care
1966	Aylett	Ileorectal anastomosis without ileostomy
1969	Kock	Kock pouch
1980	Parks and Nicholls	S-pouch
1980	Utsunomiya	J-pouch
1995	Fazio	IPAA

(pouchitis) [59]. Continent ileostomy itself, developed as a fashioned form of the reservoir, led to the "pouch" concept and gave rise to the procedure of ileal pouch-anal anastomosis (IPAA) of the 1980s.

1.5.2.2 Ileoanal-anastomosis and IPAA

Ileoanal anastomosis has naturally evolved as a procedure for eliminating rectal disease in UC while maintaining intestinal continuity and preserving anal continence. A sort of gross ileoanal anastomosis was attempted as early as 1900 but functional outcome was very poor [60]. The first official attempt at the procedure was performed by Dr. Rudolph Nissen (1896–1981), a pioneer surgeon of his years, today remembered for the development of esophageal surgery (laparoscopic Nissen fundoplication). In 1933, Nissen performed a total proctocolectomy with ileoanal anastomosis on a 10-year-old child with polyposis and reported great postoperative results [61].

In 1947, Mark Ravitch (1910–1989) and David Sabiston at Johns Hopkins Hospital, executed "anal ileostomies", first in dogs and later in two patients with UC, describing very successful results. Ravitch was an innovator, introducing mucosectomy to the surgical management of UC. He performed mucosal stripping from the remnant rectum, leaving a 2–3-inch long rectal muscular cuff [62]. In the early 1960s, he was one of the first American surgeons to introduce mechanical stapling devices, first developed in Europe, for surgical use in the United States.

In 1951, John Cedric Goligher (1912–1998) of Leeds developed the loop ileostomy to protect the healing ileoanal anastomosis [63].

In a Journal of the American Medical Association (JAMA) paper of 1952, Dr. Russell Best reviewed the literature on patients undergoing colectomy with ileo-anal anastomosis and reported that, despite the overall feasibility of the operation, there were numerous complications, particularly sepsis and anastomotic leaks. He also noted that bowel function improved over time as the distal ileum dilated [64].

In 1955, in order to reduce stool frequency and avoid fluid imbalance, Miguel A. Valiente and Harry E. Bacon performed a triple-limbed ileal pouch combined with an ileoanal anastomosis on seven dogs. Five dogs died, but two had satisfactory results, sphincter control preserved with low stool frequency, formed consistency and minimal perineal irritation [65].

In the 1970s–1980s, Sir Alan Guyatt Parks (1920–1982) and Ralph John Nicholls (b. 1943) from St. Mark's Hospital reported their experience with 21 patients who were treated with an ileal-reservoir anal anastomosis for both UC and familial polyposis. Parks' version of the ileal-reservoir consisted of the S-pouch, sutured to a denudated anus (mucosectomy was performed), with a temporary loop ileostomy. His patients had a 70% complication rate which soon decreased to about 20%. Ninety percent of patients had no trouble with mucus leakage, and they were all continent [66].

About the same time, J. Utsunomiya at the Tokyo Medical and Dental University described different types of anastomosis, each having a temporary loop ileostomy. However, the J-shaped reservoir rapidly gained favor due to its simpler construction and its favorable functional outcome, including spontaneous evacuation of the neorectum [67].

The 1980s showed great promise for the ileal pouch-anal anastomosis. With a better understanding of the rectal anatomy and improvement in surgical staplers, great progress was made in treating UC. Surgical staplers, in particular, permitted easier and faster transanal anastomosis (double-stapled technique), thus avoiding the need for mucosectomy; the procedure became more accessible for dedicated surgeons and began to spread worldwide.

A significant milestone in restorative proctocolectomy with IPAA was Dr. Victor Warren Fazio (1940–2015) from Cleveland Clinic Foundation's description of 1005 patients who underwent double-stapled J-pouch surgery.

In 1995, Fazio and his team found that even though early (such as small bowel obstruction, wound infection, pouch abscess and pouch bleeding) and late (such as pouchitis and anal stricture) complications were common, restorative proctocolectomy with an IPAA was a safe procedure, with low mortality. Although the total morbidity rate was appreciable, functional results were generally good and patient satisfaction was high. Therefore, the operation was considered successful and safe for the majority of patients and represented the gold standard for the surgical treatment of UC [68].

1.5.3   Knowledge of Ulcerative Colitis in Italy

Studies on UC in European countries (especially in Britain) during the 1950s aroused great interest and led to vast literature. At the same time in Italy, there were only a few limited contributions. In 1958, for the first time in Italy, Professor G. Placitelli of Bologna gave a lecture on UC in Genova for the Italian Surgical Society (SIC). Medical and surgical interest in UC grew rapidly in Italy, Bologna being the main school in this subject [69] (Fig. 1.1).

1.6   Ulcerative Colitis Therapy in the Modern Era (2000s–today)

A major evolution in medicine in the last 20 years has been the application of molecular biology and genetics to the understanding of disease. The massive amount of data serves as a testament to its complexity and ever-elusive etiology. Molecular techniques have revealed that cytokine tumor necrosis factor-alpha (TNF-α) plays a role in the IBD inflammatory process. Thus, anti-TNF-α

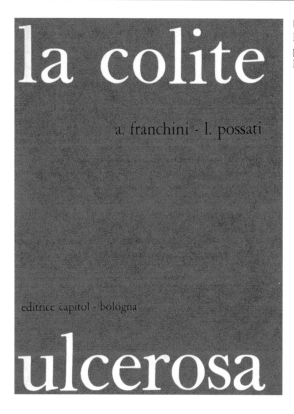

Fig 1.1 Cover of the pioneering Italian book on ulcerative colitis published by Franchini and Possati in Bologna in 1960 [69]

monoclonal antibodies have been developed to inhibit the action of TNF-α.

The first anti-TNF approved by the Food and Drug Administration (FDA) for the treatment of UC in 2005 was infliximab [70], a chimeric monoclonal antibody biologic drug which proved to be an effective alternative treatment option for patients with moderate to severe disease who had had an inadequate response to conventional glucocorticoid treatment.

In September 2012, the FDA expanded the approved use of adalimumab for the treatment of moderate-to-severe UC in adults. Adalimumab is a fully human IgG1 monoclonal antibody directed against TNF-α, administered subcutaneously. The ULTRA 2 trial confirmed the efficacy of adalimumab (induction dose 160 mg/80 mg at week 0 and week 2, followed by 40 mg every other week) for both induction and maintenance of remission [71].

The PURSUIT-SC and PURSUIT-maintenance trials introduced a third anti-TNF agent exclusively for the treatment of UC: golimumab [72], which received approval from the FDA in 2013.

Vedolizumab, a humanized monoclonal antibody directed against the α4β7 integrin, has recently entered the market as the first anti-integrin biological for the treatment of UC.

The GEMINI 1 study has evaluated the efficacy of vedolizumab for the induction and maintenance of remission in active disease. The results of the trial were impressively positive, even in the anti-TNF-experienced subgroup [73].

References

1. Kornbluth A, Sachar DB; Practice Parameters Committee of the American College of Gastroenterology (2010) Ulcerative colitis practice guidelines in adults: American College of Gastroenterology, Practice Parameters Committee. Am J Gastroenterol 105(3):501–523
2. Molodecky NA, Soon IS, Rabi DM et al (2012) Increasing incidence and prevalence of the inflammatory bowel diseases with time, based on systematic review. Gastroenterology 142(1):46–54
3. Danese S, Fiocchi C (2011) Ulcerative colitis. N Engl J Med 365(18):1713–1725
4. Molodecky NA, Kaplan GG (2010) Environmental risk factors for inflammatory bowel disease. Gastroenterol Hepatol 6(5):339–346
5. Roberts CJ, Diggle R (1982) Non-smoking: a feature of ulcerative colitis. Br Med J (Clin Res Ed) 285(6339):440
6. Rutgeerts P, D'Haens G, Hiele M et al (1994) Appendectomy protects against ulcerative colitis. Gastroenterology 106(5):1251–1253
7. Bonen DK, Cho JH (2003) The genetics of inflammatory bowel disease. Gastroenterology 124(2):521–536
8. Kirsner JB (2001) Ulcerative colitis. In: Kirsner JB, Origin and directions of inflammatory bowel disease. Kluwer Academic, Dordrecht
9. Lim ML, Wallace MR (2004) Infectious diarrhea in history. Infect Dis Clin North Am 18(2):261–274
10. Aretaeus (1856) The extant works of Aretaeus, the Cappadocian. Edited and translated by Francis Adams. London. (Republished by Milford House Inc, Boston, 1972)
11. Wilson PJE (1961) The young pretender. Br Med J 2:1226
12. Sydenham T (1701) The whole works of that excellent practical physician, Dr Thomas Sydenham, the third edition corrected from original Latin by John Pechey. Wellington, London
13. Burch W, Gump DW, Krawitt EL (1992) Historical case report of Sir William Johnson, the Mohawk Baronet. Am J Gastroenterol 87(8):1023–1025
14. Baillie M (1793) The morbid anatomy of some of the most important parts of the human body. J. Johnson and G. Nicol, London.
15. Wilks S (1859) Morbid appearances in the intestine of Miss Bankes. London Medical Gazette 2:264–265
16. Wilks S, Moxon W (1875) Lectures on pathological anatomy, 2nd edn. Lindsay and Blakiston, Philadelphia
17. Allchin WH (1909) A discussion on "ulcerative colitis": introductory address. Proc R Soc Med 2 (Med Sect):59–75
18. Mayo Robson AW (1893) Cases of colitis with ulceration treated by inguinal colostomy and local treatment of the ulcerated surfaces with subsequent closure of the artificial anus. Trans Clin Soc Lond 26:213–215
19. Weir RF (1902) A new use for the useless appendix in the surgical treatment of obstinate colitis. Med Rec (NY) 62:201–202
20. Kirsner JB (1990) The development of American gastroenterology. Raven Press, New York
21. Mulder DJ, Noble AJ, Justinich CJ, Duffin JM (2014) A tale of two diseases: the history of inflammatory bowel disease. J Crohns Colitis 8(5):341–348

22. Bassler A (1913) Ulcerative colitis. Interstate Med J 20:705–706
23. Helmholz HF (1923) Chronic ulcerative colitis in childhood. Am J Dis Child 26(5):418–430
24. Jackman RJ, Bargen JA, Helmholz HF (1940) Life histories of ninety-five children with chronic ulcerative colitis: a statistical study based on comparison with a whole group of eight hundred and seventy-one patients. Am J Dis Child 59(3):459–467
25. Davidson M (1939) Infantilism in ulcerative colitis. Arch Intern Med (Chic) 64(6):1187–1195
26. Kirsner JB, Spencer JA (1963) Family occurrences of ulcerative colitis, regional enteritis, and ileocolitis. Ann Intern Med 59:133–144
27. Hewitt JH, Howard WT (1915) Chronic ulcerative colitis with polyps: a consideration of the so called colitis polyposa (Virchow). Arch Intern Med (Chic) XV (5_1):714–723
28. Wangensteen OH, Toon RW (1948) Primary resection of the colon and rectum with particular reference to cancer and ulcerative colitis. Am J Surg 75(2):384–404
29. Gill AM (1946) Treatment of ulcerative colitis with intestinal mucosa. Proc R Soc Med 39:517–519
30. Burnford J (1930) Ulcerative colitis: its treatment by ionization: summary of twenty-eight cases. Br Med J 2(3641):640–641
31. Strauß H (1923) Ueber Kolitis-Probleme. Dtsch Med Wochenschr 49(52):1568–1570
32. Kirsner JB (2001) Historical origins of current IBD concepts. World J Gastroenterol 7(2):175–184
33. Neumann H (1943) Treatment of chronic ulcerative colitis by pneumoperitoneum. Br Med J 1(4278):9–10
34. Dennis C, Eddy FD (1947) Evaluation of vagotomy in chronic, non-specific ulcerative colitis. Proc Soc Exp Biol Med 65(2):306
35. Brown JY (1913) Value of complete physiological rest of large bowel in treatment of certain ulcerations and obstetrical lesions of this organ. Surg Gynecol Obstet 16:610–616
36. Corbett RS (1945) A review of the surgical treatment of chronic ulcerative colitis. Proc R Soc Med 38(6):277–290
37. Brooke BN (1952) The management of an ileostomy, including its complications. Lancet 2(6725):102–104
38. Turnbull RB Jr (1953) Management of the ileostomy. Am J Surg 86(5):617–624
39. Lilienthal H (1903) Extirpation of the entire colon, the upper portion of the sigmoid flexure, and four inches of the ileum for hyperplastic colitis. Ann Surg 37:616–617
40. Devine H (1943) A method of colectomy for desperate cases of ulcerative colitis. Surg Gynecol Obstet 76:136–138
41. Strauss AA, Strauss SF (1944) Surgical treatment of ulcerative colitis. Surg Clin N Am 24:211–224
42. Gardner CM, Miller GG (1951) Total colectomy for ulcerative colitis. AMA Arch Surg 63(3):370–372
43. Devine H, Devine J (1948) Subtotal colectomy and colectomy in ulcerative colitis. Br Med J 2(4567):127–131
44. Aylett SO (1966) Three hundred cases of diffuse ulcerative colitis treated by total colectomy and ileo-rectal anastomosis. Br Med J 1(5494):1001–1005
45. Parc YR, Radice E, Dozois RR (1999) Surgery for ulcerative colitis: historical perspective. A century of surgical innovations and refinements. Dis Colon Rectum 42(3):299–306
46. Svartz N (1942) Salazopyrin, a new sulfanilamide preparation. A. Therapeutic results in rheumatic polyarthritis. B. Therapeutic results in ulcerative colitis. C. Toxic manifestations in treatment with sulfanilamide preparations. Acta Med Scand 110(6):577–598
47. Svartz N (1948) The treatment of 124 cases of ulcerative colitis with salazopyrine. Attempts of desensibilization in cases of hypersensitiveness to sulfa. Acta Med Scand 130(Suppl 206):465–472
48. Baron JH, Connell AM, Lennard-Jones JE, Avery Jones F (1962) Sulphasalazine and salicylazosulphadimidine in ulcerative colitis. Lancet 279(7239):1094–1096

49. Azad Khan AK, Piris J, Truelove SC (1977) An experiment to determine the active therapeutic moiety of sulphasalazine. Lancet 310(8044):892–895

50. Campieri M, Lanfranchi GA, Bazzocchi G et al (1981) Treatment of ulcerative colitis with high-dose 5-aminosalicylic acid enemas. Lancet 318(8241):270–271

51. Caprilli R, Cesarini M, Angelucci E, Frieri G (2009) The long journey of salicylates in ulcerative colitis: the past and the future. J Crohns Colitis 3(3):149–156

52. Palmer WL, Kirsner JB (1954) Observations on the influence of corticotropins upon the course of chronic ulcerative colitis. Trans Am Clin Climatol Assoc 66:10–17

53. Truelove SC, Witts LJ (1955) Cortisone in ulcerative colitis: final report on a therapeutic trial. Br Med J 2(4947):1041–1048

54. Lennard-Jones JE, Baron JH, Connell AM, Avery Jones F (1962) A double blind controlled trial of prednisolone-21-phosphate suppositories in the treatment of idiopathic proctitis. Gut 3:207–210

55. Truelove SC, Jewell DP (1974) Intensive intravenous regimen for severe attacks of ulcerative colitis. Lancet 1(7866):1067–1070

56. Bean RH (1962) The treatment of chronic ulcerative colitis with 6-mercaptopurine. Med J Aust 49(2):592–593

57. Jewell DP, Truelove SC (1974) Azathioprine in ulcerative colitis: final report on a controlled therapeutic trial. Br Med J 4(5945):627–630

58. Lichtiger S, Present DH, Kornbluth A et al (1994) Cyclosporine in severe ulcerative colitis refractory to steroid therapy. N Engl J Med 330(26):1841–1845

59. Kock NG (1969) Intra-abdominal "reservoir" in patients with permanent ileostomy. Preliminary observations on a procedure resulting in fecal "continence" in five ileostomy patients. Arch Surg 99(2):223–231

60. Hochenegg J (1900) Meine Operationserfolge bei Rectumcarcinom. Wien Klin Wochenschr 13:399–404

61. Nissen R (1933) Demonstrationen aus der operativen Chirurgie. Zunächst einige Beobachtungen aus der plastischen Chirurgie. Zentralbl Chir 60:883

62. Ravitch M, Sabiston DC Jr (1947) Anal ileostomy with preservation of the sphincter; a proposed operation in patients requiring total colectomy for benign lesions. Surg Gynecol Obstet 84(6):1095–1099

63. Goligher JC (1951) The functional results after sphincter-saving resections of the rectum. Ann R Coll Surg Engl 8(6):421–438

64. Best RR (1952) Evaluation of ileoproctostomy to avoid ileostomy in various colon lesions. J Am Med Assoc 150(7):637–642

65. Valiente MA, Bacon HE (1955) Construction of pouch using "pantaloon" technic for pull-through of ileum following total colectomy. Am J Surg 90(5):742–750

66. Parks AG, Nicholls RJ, Belliveau P (1980) Proctocolectomy with ileal reservoir and anal anastomosis. Br J Surg 67(8):533–538

67. Utsunomiya J, Iwama T, Imajo M et al (1980) Total colectomy, mucosal proctectomy, and ileoanal anastomosis. Dis Colon Rectum 23(7):459–466

68. Fazio VW, Ziv Y, Church JM et al (1995) Ileal pouch-anal anastomoses complications and function in 1005 patients. Ann Surg 222(2):120–127

69. Franchini A, Possati L (1960) La colite ulcerosa. Editrice Capitol, Bologna

70. Sands BE, Tremaine WJ, Sandborn WJ et al (2001) Infliximab in the treatment of severe, steroid-refractory ulcerative colitis: a pilot study. Inflamm Bowel Dis 7(2):83–88

71. Sandborn WJ, van Assche G, Reinisch W et al (2012) Adalimumab induces and maintains clinical remission in patients with moderate-to-severe ulcerative colitis. Gastroenterology 142(2):257–265

72. Sandborn WJ, Feagan BG, Marano C et al (2014) Subcutaneous golimumab induces clinical response and remission in patients with moderate-to-severe ulcerative colitis. Gastroenterology 146(1):85–95

73. Feagan BG, Rutgeerts P, Sands BE et al (2013) Vedolizumab as induction and maintenance therapy for ulcerative colitis. N Engl J Med 369(8):699–710

Presentation and Natural Course of Ulcerative Colitis

2

Gilberto Poggioli and Nicola Renzi

2.1 Introduction

Ulcerative colitis (UC) is a chronic, disabling inflammatory bowel disease (IBD) which generally begins in young adulthood and lasts throughout life. It represents approximately 55% of IBD, followed by Crohn's disease (CD) and inflammatory bowel disease unclassified, and it is observed predominantly in developed countries. The clinical course is unpredictable, marked by alternating periods of exacerbation and remission. Bloody diarrhea is the characteristic symptom of the disease [1].

Its precise etiology is unknown, but it has been scientifically verified that genetic, environmental and intestinal microbial factors play an important role in the development of IBD. In fact, in recent decades, there has been an increase in knowledge regarding disease pathophysiology and a deep understanding of the complex interaction between these factors which result in mucosal inflammation.

Inflammation in UC is characteristically restricted to the mucosal surface. The disease starts in the rectum and generally extends proximally in a continuous manner through the entire colon; however, some patients with proctitis or left-sided colitis might have a cecal patch of inflammation.

Although its incidence and prevalence have stabilized in high incidence areas, such as Western Europe and North America, its incidence continues to rise in areas, such as Eastern Europe, Asia and much of the developing world [2].

In addition to significantly impacting quality of life and work productivity due to its debilitating symptoms, UC is also associated with an increased risk of colorectal cancer.

N. Renzi (✉)
Department of Medical and Surgical Sciences, University of Bologna, S. Orsola-Malpighi Hospital
Bologna, Italy
e-mail: nicola.renzi4@unibo.it

G. Poggioli (Ed), *Ulcerative Colitis*,
Updates in Surgery
DOI: 10.1007/978-88-470-3977-3_2, © Springer-Verlag Italia 2019

2.2   Definition and Classification

Ulcerative colitis is a lifelong, chronic, disabling inflammatory condition which causes continuous mucosal inflammation of the colon and rectum, not related to an intestinal infection or the use of nonsteroidal anti-inflammatory drugs. The inflammation is characterized by superficial ulcerations, granularity and a distorted vascular pattern; histological features include an expansion of the lamina propria with inflammatory cells and crypt abscesses and there are usually no fistulas or granulomas (typical histological findings of CD). The inflammation is characterized by a relapsing and remitting course, always affecting the rectum and can extend, in a proximal and continuous fashion, to other parts of the colon [3].

Inflammatory bowel disease unclassified is the definition of a small group of cases in which a well-defined distinction between UC, CD or other causes of colitis cannot be made; similarly, *indeterminate colitis* is a term used by pathologists to describe a colectomy specimen with overlapping features of UC and CD. In these cases, a definitive diagnosis can be obtained only after taking into account the history, endoscopic appearance, histopathology of multiple mucosal biopsies and appropriate radiology [4].

Endoscopy usually defines the extent of the disease, but biopsies are often necessary to determine the full extent of the colonic inflammation: the macroscopic aspect can underestimate involvement. *Ulcerative proctitis* or *proctosigmoiditis* refers to an inflammation limited to the rectum or rectosigmoid junction; *left-sided colitis* refers to inflammation extending up to, but not beyond, the splenic flexure; *extensive colitis* extends proximally to the splenic flexure or involves the right colon *(pancolitis)*. Generally, approximately half of the patients present with proctosigmoiditis, 30% with left-sided colitis and 20% with pancolitis, but a high percentage of patients with limited inflammation progress to more extensive disease (proximal extension) in adults [4].

Colitis activity can be scored using different indices, but none have been validated; in addition, flexible sigmoidoscopy and biopsy are commonly used to confirm and assess disease activity, clinical features (such as bloody stool, stool frequency, body temperature and heart rate) and laboratory markers (i.e., acute phase C-reactive protein, erythrocyte sedimentation rate, serum procalcitonin and albumin levels, fecal calprotectin and lactoferrin) are considered markers of severity [5]. It must be considered, however, that none of these markers is specific for UC, since they merely represent active inflammation.

Remission is defined as a stool frequency of ≤ 3/day, no rectal bleeding and normal mucosa at endoscopy [4].

2.3 Epidemiology and Risk Factors

2.3.1 Epidemiology

The prevalence and incidence of IBD in adult and pediatric populations have increased worldwide in recent decades, showing lower incidence in developing countries. The differences in incidence between westernized countries and developing countries have previously been explained by lower disease awareness, genetics and environmental factors. Thus, the incidence of IBD in newly industrialized countries has also rapidly increased in recent decades. The incidence of UC is higher in developed countries than in developing countries; in the same way, UC is more frequently diagnosed in urban areas than in rural areas. These findings could be partly explained by increased access to health care and better medical records in more developed than less developed countries and areas.

Ulcerative colitis has a higher incidence and prevalence in North America, northern Europe and Australia, and a north-south gradient exists, with higher incidence rates in higher latitudes [2].

The incidence of UC in the world varies from 9 to 20 cases per 100,000 people/year, ranging from 11.3 to 14.0 per 100,000 people/year in Europe based on data from prospective inception cohorts. Analogous studies have reported the highest worldwide incidence of IBD in the Faroe Islands: 83 per 100,000 people/year (with an incidence of 31.8 per 100,000 people/year in 2010 and 57.9 per 100,000 people/year in 2011 as regards UC); this result was later confirmed by a retrospective study which found similar data. These extreme values seem to be a new phenomenon in the Faroe Islands, and the cause is not yet fully understood. The UC world prevalence rates range from 156 to 291 cases per 100,000 people, and the rates are lowest in the southern hemisphere and eastern countries [2, 6–8].

Ulcerative colitis has a bimodal pattern of incidence according to age [9]. The peak age-specific incidence occurs at approximately 20 years of age (between 15 and 30 years of age), and a second smaller peak occurs at approximately 50 years of age (between 50 and 70 years of age).

2.3.2 Risk Factors

Studies have noted either no preference regarding sex or a slight predilection for men. In the United States, males and females are equally affected, but both whites and Ashkenazi Jews are at much higher risk of developing inflammatory bowel disease than the general population [10]. A family history of inflammatory bowel disease is the most important independent risk factor. The risk is particularly high in first-degree relatives [11].

Ulcerative colitis patients are most often never-smokers or non-smokers: cigarette smoking acts as a protective factor, much more than others. A meta-analysis showed that smoking is protective against UC as compared with non-smoking [12]. Patients with UC who smoke tend to have milder disease course than do non-smokers, and disease activity is often increased in those who stop smoking [13]. Another protective factor which plays an important role is, for unknown reasons, a history of appendectomy. Appendectomy is protective against UC, with the effect mainly limited to patients having had acute appendicitis before age 20 years of age [14]. A meta-analysis showed that appendectomy reduced the risk of developing UC by 69% [15]. Breastfeeding for more than 3 months, is also protective against subsequent development of UC [16]. Conversely, previous episodes of gastrointestinal infection and exposure to non-steroidal anti-inflammatory drugs represent risk factors for onset or relapse of disease.

2.4   Pathogenesis

Although the pathogenesis of IBD remains elusive, it is thought to be the result of a dysregulated immune response to gut microbiota in a genetically predisposed host, arising at a confluence of host genetic and external environmental influences. Considering, among other things, that the rapid rise in incidence in regions undergoing urbanization (westernization) and migration from a low-incidence to a high-incidence region results in an increase in the risk of IBD in the second generation, external environment plays a pivotal role. On the other hand, having an affected family member represents the strongest risk factor for developing IBD and some ethnic groups (see Ashkenazi Jews) have a rate of UC which is 3 to 5 times higher; all this supports the important role of genetic factors. Genetic studies have led to the discovery of several susceptibility genes for UC, mostly associations within the specific human leukocyte antigen (HLA) haplotype. More than 47 susceptibility loci have been associated with UC, including 20 which overlap with CD [17].

Normally, the intestinal immune system maintains equilibrium between tolerance to commensal flora and dietary antigens, and adequate responsiveness to enteric pathogens. In UC, damage to the epithelial barrier leads to increased permeability, possibly due to the defective regulation of tight junctions and alteration of the synthesis of some colonic mucin subtypes. This barrier loss enables increased uptake of luminal antigens [18]. The lamina propria is populated by macrophages and dendritic cells presenting antigens to lymphocytes (B cells and T cells), which leads to the activation of adaptive immune responses. In patients with UC, numbers of activated and mature dendritic cells are increased with increased stimulatory capacity. This could play a role in altering susceptibility to enteric infections or to changing the ability of the adaptive immune response to become tolerant to commensal bacteria. In this way, UC seems to result from a breakdown of the homeostatic balance between the host's mucosal immunity and the enteric microbiota, which results in an altered immune response against commensal non-pathogenic bacteria [19].

In particular, the altered function of regulatory and effector T-cells in UC leads to an atypical Th2 response, mediated by natural killer T-cells, which produces interleukin 13, which is of particular importance in its cytotoxic functions against epithelial cells, in apoptosis induction and in alteration of the protein composition of tight junctions [18, 20]. Natural killer T-cells are increased in the lamina propria of an inflamed colon and are capable of producing many Th2 cytokines which support the activity of natural killer T-cells themselves, amplifying tissue injury [21].

Furthermore, amplification of the inflammatory response is achieved by chemoattractants and by proinflammatory cytokines which upregulate the expression of adhesion molecules on the vascular endothelium of mucosal blood vessels. Adhesion molecules and chemoattractants recruit circulating leucocytes from the systemic circulation to the inflamed mucosa by means of adhesion and extravasation into the tissue, thus perpetuating the inflammation [22]. Antibodies against the ligands of these adhesion molecules (vedolizumab) prevent lymphocyte recruitment and reduce the severity of colonic inflammation.

Another important inflammatory mediator in pathogenesis is tumor necrosis factor-alfa (TNF-alfa), always found elevated in the blood and in the mucosa of patients with UC [23]. This important fact is supported by the effectiveness of anti-TNF treatment for the disease (infliximab, adalimumab).

2.5   Clinical Features, Complications and Diagnosis

2.5.1   Clinical Features

The diagnosis of UC is based on clinical symptoms and confirmed by objective findings from endoscopic and histological examinations. Since these features are not specific for UC, establishing the diagnosis also requires the exclusion of other causes of colitis by history, laboratory studies and by biopsies of the colon obtained on endoscopy.

Patients with UC usually present with diarrhea which may be associated with blood. Bowel movements are frequent and small in volume as a result of rectal inflammation. Associated symptoms include colicky abdominal pain, urgency, tenesmus and incontinence. The onset of symptoms is usually gradual, and symptoms are progressive over several weeks. The severity of symptoms may range from mild disease to severe disease with more than 10 stools per day with severe abdominal pain and bleeding. In clinically moderate to severe intestinal disease, systemic symptoms may be present: fever, fatigue and weight loss are the most common. Patients may also have dyspnea and palpitations due to anemia secondary to iron deficiency, blood loss, anemia from chronic disease, or autoimmune hemolytic anemia.

At physical examination, UC patients often seem normal, especially in mild cases of disease. Moderate-to-severe cases may present abdominal tenderness to palpation, fever, hypotension, tachycardia and pallor. Rectal examination may reveal evidence of blood. Patients with severe colitis and patients with prolonged diarrhea may have signs of malnutrition with muscle wasting, loss of subcutaneous fat, peripheral edema and weight loss. Most patients with UC present with an attack of mild severity at presentation, approximately one-third of patients have moderate disease, and very few patients have severe disease at presentation.

Disease activity can be objectively measured using a clinical disease activity index. The Montreal classification of the severity of UC is one such index which stratifies severity into mild, moderate, and severe [24]. Severity according to the Montreal classification is based on the number of daily stools and the presence (or absence) of systemic signs of inflammation, such as fever and tachycardia, or laboratory abnormalities. The severity of disease in patients with UC is important in clinical management and can predict long-term outcomes; in this way, it must also consider the extent of the disease (Table 2.1).

In severe UC, laboratory tests may present anemia, an elevated erythrocyte sedimentation rate ($\geq$30 mm/hour), low albumin, and electrolyte abnormalities due to diarrhea and dehydration; if primary sclerosing cholangitis is present at the same time, patients may have an elevation in serum alkaline phosphatase concentration. Due to intestinal inflammation, fecal calprotectin or lactoferrin may be elevated [5].

Table 2.1 Montreal classification of disease severity in ulcerative colitis [24]

E1	**ulcerative proctitis** (limited to the rectum or rectosigmoid junction)
E2	**left-sided UC** (distal to the splenic flexure of the colon)
E3	**extensive UC or pancolitis** (involvement proximal to the splenic flexure)
Clinical remission	No symptoms
Mild	Passage of four or fewer stools per day (with or without blood), absence of any systemic illness and normal inflammatory markers (ESR)
Moderate	Passage of more than four stools per day, but with minimal signs of systemic toxicity
Severe	Passage of at least six bloody stools daily, pulse rate of at least 90 beats/min, temperature of at least 37.5°C, hemoglobin of less than 10.5 g/dL and ESR of at least 30 mm/h

UC, ulcerative colitis; *ESR*, erythrocyte sedimentation rate

2.5.2   Acute Complications

Acute complications of the disease are possible: toxic megacolon and fulminant colitis, severe bleeding and perforation. Patients with UC may develop fulminant colitis with more than 10 stools per day, continuous bleeding, abdominal pain, distension, fever and anorexia. Patients with fulminant colitis are at high risk of developing toxic megacolon as the inflammatory process extends beyond the mucosa to involve the muscle layers of the colon and gives severe systemic toxic symptoms. Toxic megacolon is characterized by a colonic diameter ≥6 cm or a cecal diameter >9 cm, and the presence of systemic toxicity. Bleeding may also be severe in a considerable percentage of patients. Massive hemorrhage rarely occurs with UC but may necessitate urgent colectomy. Perforation of the colon most commonly occurs as a consequence of toxic megacolon or as a iatrogenic injury during endoscopy. However, it may also occur in patients during their first episode of UC due to a lack of scarring from prior attacks of colitis. Perforation with peritonitis has been associated with a high percentage of mortality in patients with UC and requires urgent colectomy.

2.5.3   Diagnosis

Although radiology is not required for the diagnosis of UC, imaging has to be performed in patients who present symptoms and to prevent complications (toxic megacolon and perforation). Abdominal radiography is usually normal in patients with mild-to-moderate disease, but may identify proximal constipation, mucosal thickening secondary to edema, or colonic dilation in patients with severe or fulminant UC. Double contrast barium enema (contraindicated in patients who are severely ill since perforation and precipitate ileus with toxic megacolon are a risk) may be normal in mild UC. Findings on barium enema may include a diffusely reticulated pattern with spiculated image collections of barium in microulcerations. In more severe disease, there may deeper ulcers, shortening of the colon, loss of haustra, narrowing of the luminal caliber, pseudopolyps, and filiform polyps. Computed tomography (CT) and magnetic resonance (MR) imaging may demonstrate marked thickening of the bowel wall, although this is not so specific for UC. In the same way, ultrasound with Doppler may demonstrate a thickened hypoechoic mucosal layer in patients with active UC. More severe cases may be associated with transmural bowel wall thickening.

Endoscopy and biopsy represent essential instrumental examinations for the diagnosis, evaluation and follow-up of the disease. Colonoscopy should also be avoided in hospitalized patients with severe colitis because of the great potential for perforation and precipitating toxic megacolon; in such patients, a flexible sigmoidoscopy should be performed and the evaluation should be limited to the rectum and distal sigmoid colon. Biopsies of the colon obtained on endoscopy are necessary to establish the chronicity of inflammation and to exclude other causes of colitis. An ileocolonoscopy allows evaluating the terminal ileum for inflammation, which would be suggestive of CD, and determining the endoscopic extent and severity of colonic disease. Inflammation generally starts in the rectum and extends proximally, in an uninterrupted pattern, involving part of, or the entire, colon. However, some patients with proctitis or left-sided colitis have a "cecal patch" (focal inflammation around the appendiceal orifice which is not contiguous with disease elsewhere in the colon), and rectal sparing is sometimes observed (for the most part, related to topical medical therapy with enemas). Ileal inflammation ("backwash" ileitis) may occasionally be seen in patients with UC with active right-sided colitis. Unlike the ileitis associated with CD which is patchy, backwash ileitis associated with UC is diffuse.

In addition to these necessary instrumental exams, establishing the diagnosis of UC also requires the exclusion of other causes of colitis by evaluating the medical history of the patient. A history of risk factors for other causes of colitis should be investigated: recent travel to areas endemic for parasitic infections, such as amebiasis, recent antibiotic use predisposing to an infection with *Clostridium difficile*, factors for sexually transmitted diseases (e.g., *Neisseria gonorrhoeae* and herpes simplex virus) which may be associated with proctitis. Furthermore, atherosclerotic disease or vasculopathy are suggestive of chronic colonic ischemia. A history of abdominal/pelvic radiation and NSAID/medication exposure should be sought as these may also be associated with colitis.

Differential diagnosis includes many causes of chronic diarrhea. The most difficult differential diagnosis is that with CD involving the colon (Crohn's colitis), and which shares the same clinical presentation and sometimes similar endoscopic features as UC: ileitis, segmental enteritis, granulomas and perianal disease (fistulas and abscesses) are suggestive of CD. Other diseases presenting with chronic diarrhea are: infectious colitis, radiation colitis, diversion colitis, solitary rectal ulcer, diverticular disease and medication-associated colitis. Stool culture, serology, imaging and, for the most part, endoscopy with biopsy usually help in reaching a diagnosis.

2.6   Natural Course, Extra-intestinal Manifestations and Malignancies

2.6.1   Natural Course

Patients with UC usually present with attacks of bloody diarrhea which last from weeks to months. The clinical course of UC is characterized by alternating periods of remission and relapse. However, a small percentage of patients have chronic symptoms and are unable to achieve complete remission. Overall, patients who initially present with proctitis have a more benign disease course and frequently respond to topical therapy whereas those who present with more extensive disease require systemic therapy and have a higher risk of colectomy.

The most important factors determining disease course are anatomical extent, response to treatment and age at presentation [25]. Generally, the natural course of pediatric UC is considered to be more severe than that of older patients. Pediatric-onset UC is characterized by its widespread location at diagnosis (60% of patients have extensive colitis) [26] and a high rate of disease extension (significantly higher proximal progression rates were reported in patients with proctitis or left-sided colitis as compared with the adult-onset population) [27]. In adults with UC, extension from the initial location has been reported to be lower than in the pediatric population [28]: patients with late-onset UC have a higher likelihood of steroid-free clinical remission as compared with those with early-onset disease. Finally, UC location appears to remain stable in a large part of elderly-onset patients as compared with approximately one half of the patients in the pediatric population where extension is reported [27, 28]. The anatomical extent of mucosal inflammation is clearly an important factor in determining disease course; patients with more severe disease tend to have more extensive forms (pancolitis) than those with less severe disease. Furthermore, disease extent is an important predictor of colectomy and colorectal cancer [29, 30]. Mucosal healing in response to treatment is also important in predicting long-term clinical outcomes; it has been demonstrated that early mucosal healing as defined by the Mayo endoscopy score in patients treated with infliximab was associated with a lower risk of colectomy and a higher rate of symptomatic remission and steroid-free remission [31, 32]. Despite the often severe disease manifestations, patients with UC do not have an increased mortality risk as compared with the general population [33].

2.6.2   Extra-intestinal Manifestations

Although UC primarily involves the bowel, it is associated with manifestations in other organ systems [34]. Although a low percentage of patients with inflammatory bowel disease have an extra-intestinal manifestation at initial presentation, up to 50% of patients with IBD experience at least one extra-intestinal manifestation in their life. The patient's quality of life is adversely affected by extra-intestinal manifestations, such as primary sclerosing cholangitis or venous thromboembolism, which can be life-threatening. The majority of extra-intestinal manifestations run in parallel with intestinal disease activity, with the exception of ankylosing spondylitis and uveitis, and with uncertainty regarding primary sclerosing cholangitis and pyoderma gangrenosum. Arthropathy and arthritis are the most frequent; they consist in both peripheral and axial arthropathies and belong to the spondyloarthritis group of conditions. Although radiological diagnosis of sacroiliitis is frequent, progression to ankylosing spondylitis occurs rarely; in the axial form, HLA-B27 is often associated. These patients should be managed by rheumatologists for the specific manifestation. Other extra-intestinal manifestations often include ocular manifestation (uveitis, episcleritis, iritis and conjunctivitis) in asymptomatic patients, skin manifestations (erythema nodosum and pyoderma gangrenosum), coagulopathy (venous thromboembolism) with a high risk of deep venous thrombosis, pulmonary embolism and arterial thromboembolism in both medical and surgical patients, and hepatobiliary manifestations. IBDs have been associated with primary sclerosing cholangitis, fatty liver and autoimmune liver disease. Patients with primary sclerosing cholangitis are usually asymptomatic and identified only by an isolated elevation in the serum alkaline phosphatase concentration. Patients may present with fatigue, pruritus, fever, chills, night sweats and upper right quadrant pain. Primary sclerosis cholangitis represents a risk factor for both liver and colon cancer and requires adequate monitoring [34].

2.6.3   Chronic Complication: Malignancies

Long-term complications of UC include strictures, dysplasia and colorectal cancer (CRC). Benign strictures can occur due to repeated episodes of inflammation, edema and muscle hypertrophy. Strictures are most frequently seen in the rectosigmoid colon and may cause symptoms of obstruction. Strictures in UC should be considered malignant until proven otherwise by endoscopic evaluation with biopsy. Surgery is indicated for strictures which cause continued symptoms of obstruction or which cannot be fully evaluated to exclude malignancy.

Patients with UC are at increased risk for CRC; UC has been defined as being a risk factor of 1.7% for CRC in all IBD patients [35]. The extent of the colitis and duration of the disease are the two most important risk factors for CRC. The risk of CRC appears to be higher in patients with pancolitis than in patients with proctitis and proctosigmoiditis, regardless of the duration of disease. Other factors associated with an increased risk of CRC include endoscopic and histological severity of inflammation, presence of dysplasia, positive family history of sporadic CRC, post-inflammatory pseudopolyps, and, for the most part, the presence of primary sclerosing cholangitis [36].

Ulcerative colitis-related CRC patients were younger than those with CRC unrelated to UC. They are also more likely to have multiple neoplastic lesions, and have higher proportions of superficial-type lesions and invasive-type lesions at histology, as well as mucinous or signet-ring cell histotypes [37, 38]. All UC patients have to continue endoscopies for surveillance and treatment of colonic lesions. Proctocolectomy, with removal of the entire colon, reduces the risk of CRC, but cancer and/or de novo polyps can still develop in the anal transition zone.

References

1. Latella G, Papi C (2012) Crucial steps in the natural history of inflammatory bowel disease. World J Gastroenterol 18(29):3790–3799
2. Burisch J, Pedersen N, Čuković-Čavka S et al (2914) East-West gradient in the incidence of inflammatory bowel disease in Europe: the ECCO-EpiCom inception cohort. Gut 63(4):588–597
3. Farmer RG, Easley KA, Rankin GB (1993) Clinical patterns, natural history, and progression of ulcerative colitis: a long-term follow-up of 1116 patients. Dig Dis Sci 38(6): 1137–1146
4. Magro F, Gionchetti P, Eliakim R et al; European Crohn's and Colitis Organisation [ECCO] (2017) Third European evidence-based consensus on diagnosis and management of ulcerative colitis. Part 1: definitions, diagnosis, extra-intestinal manifestations, pregnancy, cancer surveillance, surgery, and ileo-anal pouch disorders. J Crohns Colitis 11(6):649–670
5. Sands BE (2015) Biomarkers of inflammation in inflammatory bowel disease. Gastroenterology 149(5):1275–1285
6. Loftus EV Jr, Silverstein MD, Sandborn WJ et al (2000) Ulcerative colitis in Olmsted County, Minnesota, 1940-1993: incidence, prevalence, and survival. Gut 46(3):336–343
7. Vegh Z, Burisch J, Pedersen N et al (2014) Incidence and initial disease course of inflammatory bowel diseases in 2011 in Europe and Australia: results of the 2011 ECCO-EpiCom inception cohort. J Crohns Colitis 8(11):1506–1515
8. Hammer T, Nielsen KR, Munkholm P et al (2016) The Faroese IBD Study: incidence of inflammatory bowel diseases across 54 years of population–based data. J Crohns Colitis 10(8):934–942
9. Loftus EV Jr, Sandborn WJ (2002) Epidemiology of inflammatory bowel disease. Gastroenterol Clin North Am 31(1):1–20
10. Birkenfeld S, Zvidi I, Hazazi R, Niv Y (2009) The prevalence of ulcerative colitis in Israel: a twenty-year survey. J Clin Gastroenterol 43(8):743–746
11. Orholm M, Munkholm P, Langholz E et al (1991) Familial occurrence of inflammatory bowel disease. N Engl J Med 324(2):84–88
12. Mahid SS, Minor KS, Soto RE et al (2006) Smoking and inflammatory bowel disease: a meta-analysis. Mayo Clin Proc 81(11):1462–1471
13. Beaugerie L, Massot N, Carbonnel F et al (2001) Impact of cessation of smoking on the course of ulcerative colitis. Am J Gastroenterol 96(7):2113–2116
14. Andersson RE, Olaison G, Tysk C, Ekbom A (2001) Appendectomy and protection against ulcerative colitis. N Engl J Med 344(11):808–814
15. Koutroubakis IE, Vlachonikolis IG (2000) Appendectomy and the development of ulcerative colitis: results of a meta-analysis of published case-control studies. Am J Gastroenterol 95(1):171–176
16. Klement E, Cohen RV, Boxman J et al (2004) Breastfeeding and risk of inflammatory bowel disease: a systematic review with meta-analysis. Am J Clin Nutr 80(5):1342–1352
17. Anderson CA, Boucher G, Lees CW et al (2011) Meta-analysis identifies 29 additional ulcerative colitis risk loci, increasing the number of confirmed associations to 47. Nat Genet 43(3):246–252
18. Heller F, Florian P, Bojarski C et al (2005) Interleukin-13 is the key effector Th2 cytokine in ulcerative colitis that affects epithelial tight junctions, apoptosis, and cell restitution. Gastroenterology 129(2):550–564
19. Frank DN, Robertson CE, Hamm CM et al (2011) Disease phenotype and genotype are associated with shifts in intestinal-associated microbiota in inflammatory bowel diseases. Inflamm Bowel Dis 17(1):179–184
20. Heller F, Fromm A, Gitter AH et al (2008) Epithelial apoptosis is a prominent feature of the epithelial barrier disturbance in intestinal inflammation: effect of pro-inflammatory interleukin-13 on epithelial cell function. Mucosal Immunol 1(Suppl 1):S58–S61

21. Steel AW, Mela CM, Lindsay JO et al (2011) Increased proportion of CD16(+) NK cells in the colonic lamina propria of inflammatory bowel disease patients, but not after azathioprine treatment. Aliment Pharmacol Ther 33(1):115–126
22. Briskin M, Winsor-Hines D, Shyjan A et al (1997) Human mucosal addressin cell adhesion molecule-1 is preferentially expressed in intestinal tract and associated lymphoid tissue. Am J Pathol 151(1):97–110
23. Masuda H, Iwai S, Tanaka T, Hayakawa S (1995) Expression of IL-8, TNF-alpha and IFN-gamma m-RNA in ulcerative colitis, particularly in patients with inactive phase. J Clin Lab Immunol 46(3):111–123
24. Silverberg MS, Satsangi J, Ahmad T et al (2005) Toward an integrated clinical, molecular and serological classification of inflammatory bowel disease: Report of a Working Party of the 2005 Montreal World Congress of Gastroenterology. Can J Gastroenterol 19(Suppl A):5A –36A
25. Duricova D, Burisch J, Jess T et al; ECCO-EpiCom (2014) Age-related differences in presentation and course of inflammatory bowel disease: an update on the population-based literature. J Crohns Colitis 8(11):1351–1361
26. Gower-Rousseau C, Dauchet L, Vernier-Massouille G et al (2009) The natural history of pe-diatric ulcerative colitis: a population-based cohort study. Am J Gastroenterol 104(8):2080–2088
27. Langholz E, Munkholm P, Krasilnikoff PA, Binder V (1997) Inflammatory bowel diseases with onset in childhood. Clinical features, morbidity, and mortality in a regional cohort. Scand J Gastroenterol 32(2):139–147
28. Magro F, Rodrigues A, Vieira AI et al (2012) Review of the disease course among adult ulcerative colitis population-based longitudinal cohorts. Inflamm Bowel Dis 18(3):573–583
29. Hoie O, Wolters FL, Riis L et al; European Collaborative Study Group of Inflammatory Bowel Disease (2007) Low colectomy rates in ulcerative colitis in an unselected European cohort followed for 10 years. Gastroenterology 132(2):507–515
30. Jess T, Loftus EV Jr, Velayos FS et al (2006) Risk of intestinal cancer in inflammatory bowel disease: a population-based study from Olmsted county, Minnesota. Gastroenterology 130(4):1039–1046
31. Reinisch W, Sandborn WJ, Rutgeerts P et al (2012) Long-term infliximab maintenance therapy for ulcerative colitis: the ACT-1 and ACT-2 extension studies. Inflamm Bowel Dis 18(2):201–211
32. Rutgeers P, Sandborn WJ, Feagan BG et al (2005) Infliximab for induction and maintenance therapy for ulcerative colitis. N Engl J Med 353(23):2462–2476
33. Jess T, Gamborg M, Munkholm P, Sørensen TI (2007) Overall and cause-specific mortality in ulcerative colitis: meta-analysis of population-based inception cohort studies. Am J Gastroenterol 102(3):609–617
34. Harbord M, Annese V, Vavricka SR et al; European Crohn's and Colitis Organisation [ECCO] (2016) ECCO Guideline/Consensus Paper. The First European Evidence-based Consensus on Extra-intestinal Manifestations in Inflammatory Bowel Disease. J Crohns Colitis 10(3):239–254
35. Lutgens MW, van Oijen MG, van der Heijden GJ et al (2013) Declining risk of colorectal cancer in inflammatory bowel disease: an updated meta-analysis of population-based cohort studies. Inflamm Bowel Dis 19(4):789–799
36. Annese V, Beaugerie L, Egan L et al; European Crohn's and Colitis Organisation [ECCO] (2015) European Evidence-based Consensus: Inflammatory Bowel Disease and Malignan-cies. J Crohns Colitis 9(11):945–965
37. Watanabe T, Konishi T, Kishimoto J et al (2011) Ulcerative colitis-associated colorectal cancer shows a poorer survival than sporadic colorectal cancer: a nationwide Japanese study. Inflamm Bowel Dis 17(3):802–808
38. Hrabe JE, Byrn JC, Button AM et al (2014) A matched case-control study of IBD-associated colorectal cancer: IBD portends worse outcome. J Surg Oncol 109(2):117–121

Diagnosis of Ulcerative Colitis: the Role of Imaging Techniques

3

Carla Serra, Chiara Praticò, and Alberta Cappelli

3.1 Introduction

The diagnosis of ulcerative colitis (UC) is based on a combination of endoscopic, histological, radiological and biochemical investigations.

Endoscopy, together with histology, is currently considered the diagnostic gold standard for the evaluation of disease activity and extent, and it is necessary for the surveillance of UC-related colonic cancer. Endoscopic reassessment is also appropriate at disease relapse, for steroid-dependent or refractory UC or when considering colectomy [1]. However, in cases of severe disease activity or in the presence of strictures, evaluation of the disease extent may not be feasible using conventional colonoscopy. Moreover, bowel cleansing and procedure-related discomfort are often a major cause of patient rejection of repeated colonoscopies, even more so in the case of young patients or children. Therefore, many studies have investigated a non-invasive approach for evaluating patients with UC, in both the acute and chronic setting.

While transabdominal ultrasound and magnetic resonance (MR) imaging have high accuracy for assessing the activity and severity of Crohn's colitis, its performance in UC is less clear, and the role of computed tomography (CT) for differentiating quiescent from active colonic inflammation is currently not defined [2]. All these imaging techniques give supplementary information to endoscopic assessment of disease activity, but in current guidelines and clinical practice, the resolution of radiological abnormalities is not considered a treatment endpoint in UC patients. A more defined role for imaging techniques is provided in the case of UC complications, such as abdominal radiography when toxic megacolon is suspected and CT in the case of colonic

C. Serra (✉)
Interventional Ultrasound Unit, Department of Organ Failure and Transplantation,
S. Orsola-Malpighi Hospital
Bologna, Italy
e-mail: carla.serra@aosp.bo.it

G. Poggioli (Ed), *Ulcerative Colitis*,
Updates in Surgery
DOI: 10.1007/978-88-470-3977-3_3, © Springer-Verlag Italia 2019

strictures [1]. The diagnosis of extraintestinal complications, such as primary sclerosing cholangitis, mesenteric thrombosis, nephrolithiasis, cholelithiasis and sacroiliitis, also rely on cross-sectional imaging techniques. In addition, imaging techniques play a central role in excluding the involvement of the small bowel and in ruling out the possibility of Crohn's disease (CD).

3.2   Abdominal Radiography

3.2.1   Clinical Settings

Plain abdominal radiography is indicated in an acute setting to assess the colonic dilatation. Plain films have no role in routine assessment because they cannot adequately determine the distribution of disease activity.

3.2.2   Imaging Findings

In acute severe colitis, abdominal radiography is the first study used to detect toxic megacolon which is a life-threatening complication of severe UC. It denotes a clinical syndrome characterized by systemic toxicity according to the criteria of Jalan et al. (i.e., fever, tachycardia, dehydration, altered level of consciousness, hypotension, neutrophilic leukocytosis, electrolyte disturbances), associated with evidence of colonic dilatation, defined by a mid-transverse colon luminal diameter >5.5 cm (Fig. 3.1). Toxic dilatation is the result of acute transmural inflammation and is most commonly observed in the transverse colon, the

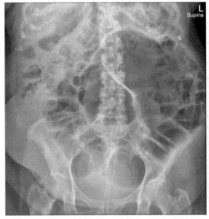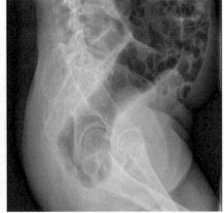

Fig. 3.1 Anteroposterior and lateral supine abdominal radiography showing abnormal distension of the colon in ulcerative colitis with toxic megacolon

most anterior portion of the colon in the supine scanning position. In addition to dilatation, the haustral folds might be edematous, giving the bowel wall a nodular contour [3–5]. Other radiological signs, such as increased small bowel gas, small bowel or gastric distension, mucosal islands (areas of preserved colonic mucosa among denuded ulcerated mucosa), colonic dilatation and deep ulceration may predict the failure of medical therapy and the development of toxic megacolon in patients with severe UC [2].

3.3   Ultrasonography

3.3.1   Clinical Settings

Ultrasonography (US) is a non-invasive, well-tolerated, radiation-free imaging technique, even though its performance is operator-dependent. In expert hands, bowel US could be a first line tool in the assessment of patients with inflammatory bowel disease (IBD). The role of US in assessing activity and extension has been widely investigated in CD affecting the small bowel, in particular the terminal ileum, and it has high accuracy in detecting stenotic and penetrating complications (fistula, abscess). When considering the colonic involvement, bowel US assessment has been shown to correlate with inflammation in CD and UC and it has been introduced into the latest ECCO guidelines as a useful tool as an adjunct to endoscopy for the diagnosis of colonic IBD [2, 6]. However, the diagnostic performance of bowel US in detecting inflammatory colonic alterations largely depends on the disease site; sensitivity is high for sigmoid/descending colonic localization while it is very low for the rectum, which is difficult to be accessed with US [7–9]. The intestinal segments involved in patients with UC are more accessible via endoscopy and, although US examination cannot replace endoscopy in the assessment of UC, it may be of use in reducing the number of diagnostic studies during follow-up.

3.3.2   Preparation

In order to reduce luminal air, it is recommended that the patient fast at least 6 hours before the examination whereas the use of a laxative is not required before routine abdominal US [10]. The scanning positions include the left and right quadrants of the upper and lower abdomen. The first evaluation with a low-frequency convex transducer (1–6 MHz) should be completed by a high-frequency (10–18 MHz) linear array probe, which increases spatial resolution and allows evaluation of the bowel wall thickness, layer pattern and bowel diameter [11].

3.3.3   Imaging Findings

Ulcerative colitis affects the rectum and extends proximally, involving the colon continuously. Therefore, the main alterations are usually detected in the left iliac fossa and in the hypogastric regions, and, in pancolitis, they extend throughout the entire colon. Rectal sparing can occur especially in the case of topical therapy. "Backwash ileitis", an inflammation of the last centimeter of the distal ileum caused by reflux of the colonic contents into the small bowel, is observed in 10–25% of patients with ulcerative pancolitis [12]. It does not present extensive ulcerations or stenosis as in CD ileitis.

The US features reflect the pathological changes of the bowel wall. The segments of the colon involved appear symmetrically and concentrically thickened (≥3 mm) and are often relatively aperistaltic (Figs. 3.2 and 3.3). The degree of thickness of the bowel wall depends on the disease activity, being higher in active disease and normal in quiescent phases. Since inflammation involves the mucosa and the superficial submucosa, bowel wall stratification is normally preserved as opposed to the segmental often lost-layering pattern of involvement in CD (Fig. 3.4) [13, 14]. A prevalent hypoechoic pattern, sometimes giving the appearance of loss of stratification, has been observed in cases of severe active UC, with swollen mucosa and edema involving the submucosa. After several recurrences, in quiescent disease and in some cases with mild inflammation, the colonic wall shows predominant hyperechoic submucosa contrasting with the hypoechoic inner mucosa, due to submucosal fat deposition (Fig. 3.5) [15]. The bowel wall can sometimes collapse and cannot be clearly delineated from the lumen, or the air trapped between the mucosal folds and ulcers can generate multiple echogenic foci without a clearly defined outer hypoechoic region [16]. In early UC, the haustral folds, normally defined as echo-poor indentations that

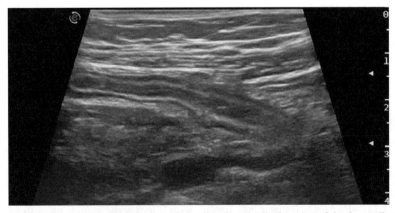

Fig. 3.2 Ultrasound findings in ulcerative colitis. Longitudinal section of the descending colon in a patient with left-sided mild active ulcerative colitis. Thickened bowel walls characterized by a stratified echo pattern and the absence of haustra coli in the relatively aperistaltic left colon

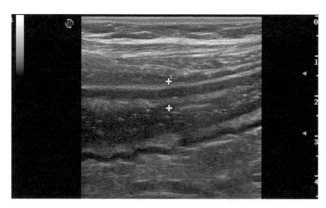

Fig. 3.3 Frequent ultrasound features of a patient with ulcerative colitis: continuous and symmetrical thickness of the bowel wall

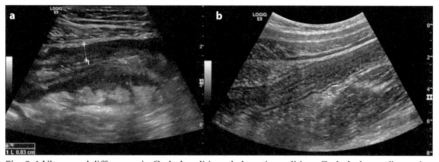

Fig. 3.4 Ultrasound differences in Crohn's colitis and ulcerative colitis. **a** Crohn's descending active colitis characterized by wall thickness, patchy loss of stratification, and initial fistulizing tracts in the bowel wall (hypoechoic spicules arising from the bowel wall and deepening in the thickened mesentery). **b**: moderate active left-sided ulcerative colitis with thickened, stratified bowel wall, having a predominant hypoechoic pattern. The loss of haustra gives a tubularized colonic shape

intersperse the colonic wall every 3–5 cm, may appear thickened as a result of inflammation and edema (Fig. 3.6). As the disease become chronic, haustra can be lost and the colon appears as a tubular structure (Fig. 3.7) [17].

Color-Doppler imaging gives additional information for assessing the inflammatory activity of UC. In cases of active UC, increased vascularization can be detected by color and power-Doppler as intramural vascular signals [18–20]. Mean blood flow volume and mean peak systolic and end diastolic velocities in the inferior mesenteric artery have been shown to be higher in patients with active rather than inactive UC [21].

3.3.4 Scoring Systems

Although the effectiveness of the studies depends on specifically experienced sonographers and might not be generalizable, the studies of Parente et al. suggest that an ultrasound score, based on bowel wall thickness and intraluminal blood

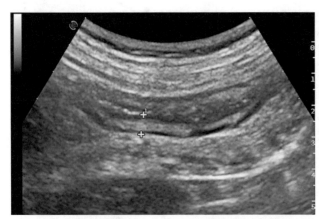

Fig. 3.5 Ultrasound findings in chronically active ulcerative colitis, showing slight thickening of the colonic wall, with predominant echogenic submucosa contrasting with the hypoechoic inner mucosa and outer muscularis propria

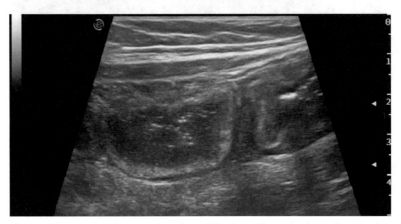

Fig. 3.6 Ultrasound findings in ulcerative colitis. Ascending colon in moderate active ulcerative pancolitis. Haustral folds appear thickened, with a stratified echo pattern

flow graded via power Doppler, can be used to assess the short-term response of severe UC to therapy and to predict disease outcomes at 15 months [8, 19]. A study in a pediatric UC population has evaluated the effectiveness of bowel US in assessing the extent and activity of disease, and the ultrasound score strongly correlated with the clinical and endoscopic activity [22].

Moreover, some studies from Limberg et al. have reported good correlations between endoscopy and the severity of colonic lesions as assessed by hydrocolonic US whereas these findings have not always been reproduced. Hydrocolonic US consists of transabdominal US after the retrograde instillation of saline solution into the colon, which may allow more detailed imaging of the bowel wall and lumen than conventional US [23, 24]. Quantitative parameters using contrast-enhanced ultrasound (CEUS) and a specific quantification software have also been proposed in a study from Girlich et al. in order to assess the histological inflammatory activity in UC, with interesting results [25].

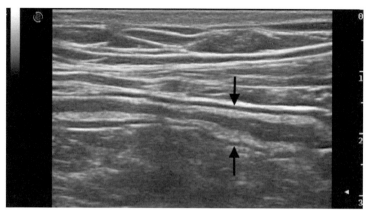

Fig. 3.7 Ultrasound findings in chronically active left-sided ulcerative colitis with a loss of haustra, a tubularized colonic shape and predominant echogenic submucosa due to submucosal fat deposition (*arrows*)

All these intriguing findings need to be additionally explored before transabdominal US can be introduced to a greater extent in the therapeutic management of UC.

3.4 Computed Tomography

3.4.1 Clinical Settings

Computed tomography enterography and colonography (virtual colonoscopy) evaluate bowel wall features by means of enteric and intravenous contrast administration. This diagnostic tool has high spatial and temporal resolution, in particular for the study of the small bowel wall, lumen and perienteric tissues. CT is associated with radiation exposure, even if the improvements in CT technology in recent years have dramatically reduced the radiation dosage.

Computed tomography enterography is indicated for the study of the small bowel in CD in order to detect disease location, activity, and inflammatory and fibrostenotic complications. In UC, the indications for CT enterography and colonography are currently restricted to colonic study in patients with strictures precluding endoscopic assessment or in patients with severe comorbidities where colonoscopy is contraindicated. It also allows excluding small bowel involvement for the differential diagnosis of CD or in the case of indeterminate colitis [1, 2, 26, 27].

Computed tomography without oral contrast is also indicated for the evaluation of toxic megacolon in equivocal or selected cases in which plain radiography does not appear to be sufficient (e.g., bowel perforation might be silent in patients taking high-dose steroids) [28, 29]. It can also be used as a primary imaging modality to screen for complications (perforation, abscess, thrombosis, ischemia) which require emergency surgery [2].

3.4.2 Preparation

Patients are required to fast for 4 hours before CT. A neutral enteric contrast agent is administered in multiple aliquots prior to the examination. Enteric contrast agents (low-contrast barium solution, sorbitol, polyethylene glycol electrolyte solution, methylcellulose solution or water) distend the lumen for a sufficient time during which images can be obtained and visualization of the bowel wall, and the inflamed bowel segments and masses is facilitated. Anti-peristaltic agents, such as glucagon or butylscopolamine, are not needed for CT enterography, thanks to the speed of imaging acquisition. Currently, the entire abdomen and pelvis can be scanned in 20 seconds or less, depending on the CT parameters.

In addition to enteric contrast, intravenous iodinated contrast is given through an intravenous catheter in order to enhance the bowel wall.

3.4.3 Imaging Findings

As in Crohn's colorectal involvement, colonic wall thickening is the most sensitive sign of bowel inflammation in UC, often accompanied by mural hyperenhancement. Unlike the patchy pattern of CD, the pattern of UC inflammation is continuous from the rectum proximally; the mesenteric and the antimesenteric colonic walls are both involved to a similar degree (Fig. 3.8).

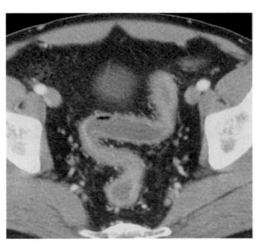

Fig. 3.8 Contrast-enhanced axial CT image showing sigmoid colon thickening and hyperenhancement in active ulcerative colitis

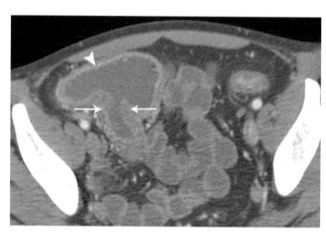

Fig. 3.9 CT enterography. Contrast-enhanced axial CT image showing backwash ileitis: patulous ileocecal valve (*arrows*) associated with mural hyperenhancement of the cecal wall (*arrowhead*)

Mild inflammation can involve the ileocecal valve when the UC extends to the cecum, and can be associated with "backwash ileitis", appearing as a patulous ileocecal valve, with mild symmetrical mural hyperenhancement of the terminal ileum (Fig. 3.9) [30]. Submucosal fat deposition is seen more commonly in UC than in Crohn's colitis, in particular in the rectum; marked rectal wall thickening can lead to luminal narrowing. Prominent perirectal fibrofatty proliferation and widening of the presacral space is also frequently observed (Fig. 3.10) [31].

As the inflammation becomes chronic, haustral folds might be lost, and colonic shortening with a tubular shape might also be seen. The exact cause of the shortening of the colon has not yet been ascertained; thinning and relaxation of the muscularis mucosae in conjunction with luminal narrowing and loss of the haustra might be a possible explanation [32]. The development of pseudopolyps (i.e., post-inflammatory polyps) is an adjunctive mark of chronic inflammation, appearing as polypoid colonic filling defects, usually enhancing on contrast-enhanced sequences (Fig. 3.11) [33].

As in plain radiography, the suspicion of toxic megacolon is demonstrated by the presence of distension of the colon, most commonly the transverse colon; the haustra appear edematous and distorted or may be absent. The presence of pneumatosis indicates ischemia and necrosis since the major complication of toxic megacolon is perforation, detected as extraluminal air at CT or radiography [34].

3.4.4   Scoring Systems

Few studies have investigated the accuracy of CT in assessing UC activity, finding a moderate correlation with endoscopic colonic inflammation (an overall sensitivity of 74%) [35, 36]. Overall, the limited data available regarding CT or CT enterography in UC does not provide adequate diagnostic performance in clinical management, and colonoscopy remains the reference standard [1, 37].

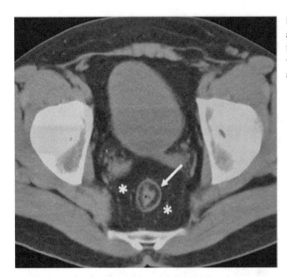

Fig. 3.10 Axial CT image showing a thickened rectum with perirectal fibrofatty proliferation and widening of the presacral space in active ulcerative colitis (*asterisks*)

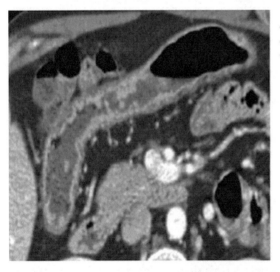

Fig. 3.11 Contrast-enhanced axial CT image showing a tubularized colon with pseudopolyps in chronically active ulcerative colitis

3.5   Magnetic Resonance Imaging

3.5.1   Clinical Settings

Similar to CT, MR imaging complements endoscopy in patients with incomplete examinations who require assessment of disease extension, and rules out small bowel involvement for the differential diagnosis of CD [38, 39]. Moreover, even if MR imaging has the best performance in evaluating the small bowel (MR enterography), it also demonstrates good sensitivity for evaluating disease activity in colonic CD and UC (MR colonography), in particular in moderate-to-severe disease [40–42].

The major disadvantages of MR enterography and colonography are longer acquisition time than CT enterography, decreased temporal and spatial resolution, and less availability of the technique. On the other hand, MR imaging has a higher contrast resolution and, most importantly, does not use ionizing radiation. In addition, a range of objective scores has been developed for MR imaging to evaluate intestinal disease activity and severity, for both UC and CD [41, 42].

3.5.2 Preparation

Patients are required to fast 4–6 hours prior to the exam or preferably overnight; for MR colonography, routine bowel cleansing, as for colonoscopy, is usually required, even if some studies adopting diffusion-weighted imaging performed the exam without preparation.

Individual protocols are tailored to the patient depending on the manufacturer and magnet strength. The majority of sequences include a combination of T1-, T2-weighted, contrast-enhanced gradient echo sequences and steady-state free precession sequences; diffusion-weighted sequences are also being increasingly introduced into the current protocols [41, 43].

Magnetic resonance colonography usually requires the supine position while, for MR enterography, patients can be studied in both a prone or a supine position. When MR colonography is performed, it is generally a part of an MR entero-colonography study and, in addition to oral contrast for small bowel evaluation, it requires colonic distension by means of a rectal enema. A warm water tap enema is administered by placing a flexible rectal catheter to infuse a water volume of 1.5–2.5 L. This allows lumen distension with a detailed assessment of the bowel wall and displaces air from the lumen-reducing artefacts. Enteric contrast agents are classified into positive, negative or biphasic, according to the effect on the signal intensity of the bowel lumen; biphasic agents are those most utilized (i.e., non-absorbable iso-osmolar solutions, such as polyethylene glycol, mannitol or methylcellulose). Water is a biphasic agent and, like the other biphasic contrast agents, it emits a variable signal intensity depending on the sequence applied (low signal intensity on T1-weighted imaging and high signal intensity on T2-weighted imaging). Anti-peristaltic agents (e.g., hyoscine N-butylbromide) can be administered before the examination to minimize peristaltic artefacts and increase colonic distension tolerance. Gadoteridol is the intravenous gadolinium-based MR contrast agent typically administered [30].

3.5.3 Imaging Findings

The rectosigmoid colon is classically involved, and the disease extends proximally; "backwash ileitis" is rare and is observed in cases of pancolitis, as previously described. As for CT imaging, the main feature is the uniform thickening of the wall, with mean values of 7–8 mm, even if, in severe disease, it can exceed 10 mm (Fig. 3.12). Wall stratification is usually maintained. The contour of the colonic wall is typically smooth and regular, as opposed to the outer mural irregularity often detected in Crohn's colitis (Fig. 3.13). As in

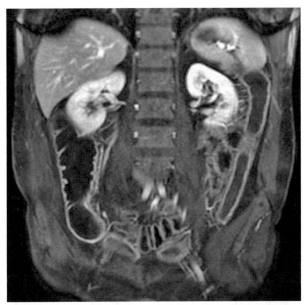

Fig. 3.12 MR enterography. Coronal contrast-enhanced T1-weighted imaging. Wall thickening and hyperenhancement of the descending colon in active ulcerative colitis

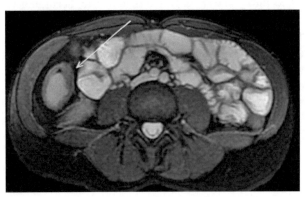

Fig. 3.13 MR enterography. Axial T2-weighted imaging. Thickening of the ascending colon in an ulcerative colitis patient (*arrow*)

CD, engorgement of the vasa recta (the so-called "comb sign") and mucosal hyperenhancement are often observed as well as pericolic fluid in cases of severe disease. Long-standing disease is characterized by wall thickening, loss of haustral folds and luminal narrowing with a typical tubular shape, apparently due to hypertrophy of the muscularis mucosa (Figs. 3.14 and 3.15). Mesenteric fatty proliferation in the perirectal space can also be well detected by MR imaging [44].

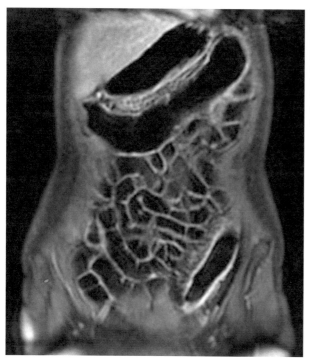

Fig. 3.14 MR enterography. Coronal contrast medium-enhanced T1-weighted imaging. Tubularized sigmoid colon and dilatation of the transverse colon in a patient with chronically active ulcerative colitis

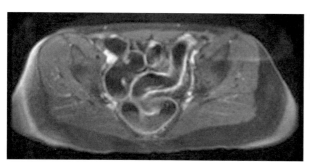

Fig. 3.15 MR enterography. Axial contrast-enhanced T1-weighted imaging. Tubularized sigmoid colon in a patient with chronically active ulcerative colitis

3.5.4   Scoring Systems

Several studies have demonstrated that MR imaging could be a valuable tool for the assessment of UC activity, reporting higher sensitivity in UC (58.8–68%) than in CD (31.6–40%), also for diffusion-weighted MR imaging. In addition, MR imaging performs better in moderate-severe UC than in mild disease [41, 45–49].

Two scoring systems have been described for the assessment of colonic inflammation in UC. A simplified MR colonography index (MRC-S), based on contrast agent uptake, the presence of edema, lymphadenopathy and comb sign, significantly correlates with endoscopy; moreover, the presence of an MRC-S ≥1 showed high sensitivity and specificity for the diagnosis of active disease (87% and 88%, respectively) [42]. The other score is based on MR diffusion-weighted imaging without any bowel preparation. Oussalah et al. showed that a segmental MR-score-S >1 had a sensitivity and specificity of 89% and 86%, respectively, when compared with endoscopic assessment of the inflammation, with higher accuracy for detecting colonic inflammation in UC than in CD [41].

These interesting results show that MR colonography can be considered an alternative to colonoscopy for the assessment and monitoring of UC activity, especially in those patients with an established diagnosis and with limitations to a completed colonoscopy or contraindications for disease severity. In addition to the above-mentioned intrinsic limitations of MR examination (i.e., availability, time and cost), it remains to be determined whether MR imaging is responsive to changes induced by treatment; therefore, colonoscopy still remains the reference standard in guiding UC management.

References

1. Magro F, Gionchetti P, Eliakim R et al; European Crohn's and Colitis Organisation [ECCO] (2017) Third European evidence-based consensus on diagnosis and management of ulcerative colitis. Part 1: Definitions, diagnosis, extra-intestinal manifestations, pregnancy, cancer surveillance, surgery, and ileo-anal pouch disorders. J Crohns Colitis 11(6):649–670
2. Panes J, Bouhnik Y, Reinisch W et al (2013) Imaging techniques for assessment of inflammatory bowel disease: joint ECCO and ESGAR evidence-based consensus guidelines. J Crohns Colitis 7(7):556–585
3. Jalan KN, Sircus W, Card WI et al (1969) An experience of ulcerative colitis. I. Toxic dilation in 55 cases. Gastroenterology 57(1):68–82
4. Benchimol EI, Turner D, Mann EH et al (2008) Toxic megacolon in children with inflammatory bowel disease: clinical and radiographic characteristics. Am J Gastroenterol 103(6):1524–1531
5. Norland CC, Kirsner JB (1969) Toxic dilatation of colon (toxic megacolon): etiology, treatment and prognosis in 42 patients. Medicine (Baltimore) 48(3):229–250
6. Pascu M, Roznowski AB, Müller HP et al (2004) Clinical relevance of transabdominal ultrasonography and magnetic resonance imaging in patients with inflammatory bowel disease of the terminal ileum and large bowel. Inflamm Bowel Dis 10(4):373–382

7. Parente F, Greco S, Molteni M et al (2003) Role of early ultrasound in detecting inflammatory intestinal disorders and identifying their anatomical location within the bowel. Aliment Pharmacol Ther 18(10):1009–1016

8. Parente F, Molteni M, Marino B et al (2010) Are colonoscopy and bowel ultrasound useful for assessing response to short-term therapy and predicting disease outcome of moderate-to-severe forms of ulcerative colitis? A prospective study. Am J Gastroenterol 105(5):1150–1157

9. Maconi G, Ardizzone S, Parente F, Bianchi Porro G (1999) Ultrasonography in the evaluation of extension, activity, and follow-up of ulcerative colitis. Scand J Gastroenterol 34(11):1103–1107

10. Pinto PN, Chojniak R, Cohen MP et al (2011) Comparison of three types of preparations for abdominal sonography. J Clin Ultrasound 39(4):203–208

11. Nylund K, Maconi G, Hollerweger A et al (2017) EFSUMB Recommendations and guidelines for gastrointestinal ultrasound. Ultraschall Med 38(3):e1–e15

12. Eisenberg RL (1996) Gastrointestinal radiology: a pattern approach. Lippincott-Raven, Philadelphia

13. Strobel D, Goertz RS, Bernatik T (2011) Diagnostics in inflammatory bowel disease: ultrasound. World J Gastroenterol 17(27):3192–3197

14. Faure C, Belarbi N, Mougenot JF et al (1997) Ultrasonographic assessment of inflammatory bowel disease in children: comparison with ileocolonoscopy. J Pediatr 130(1):147–151

15. Dietrich CF (2009) Significance of abdominal ultrasound in inflammatory bowel disease. Dig Dis 27(4):482–493

16. Khaw KT, Yeoman LJ, Saverymuttu SH et al (1991) Ultrasonic patterns in inflammatory bowel disease. Clin Radiol 43(3):171–175

17. Bartram CI, Thomson JPS, Price AB (1983) Radiology in inflammatory bowel disease. Marcel Dekker, New York

18. Heyne R, Rickes S, Bock P et al (2002) Non-invasive evaluation of activity in inflammatory bowel disease by power Doppler sonography. Z Gastroenterol 40(3):171–175

19. Parente F, Molteni M, Marino B et al (2009) Bowel ultrasound and mucosal healing in ulcerative colitis. Dig Dis 27(3):285–290

20. Parente F, Marino B, Ardizzoia A et al (2011) Impact of a population-based colorectal cancer screening program on local health services demand in Italy: a 7-year survey in a northern province. Am J Gastroenterol 106(11):1986–1993

21. Siğirci A, Baysal T, Kutlu R et al (2001) Doppler sonography of the inferior and superior mesenteric arteries in ulcerative colitis. J Clin Ultrasound 29(3):130–139

22. Civitelli F, Di Nardo G, Oliva S et al (2014) Ultrasonography of the colon in pediatric ulcerative colitis: a prospective, blind, comparative study with colonoscopy. J Pediatr 165(1):78–84

23. Limberg B, Osswald B (1994) Diagnosis and differential diagnosis of ulcerative colitis and Crohn's disease by hydrocolonic sonography. Am J Gastroenterol 89(7):1051–1057

24. Bru C, Sans M, Defelitto MM et al (2001) Hydrocolonic sonography for evaluating inflammatory bowel disease. AJR Am J Roentgenol 177(1):99–105

25. Girlich C, Schacherer D, Jung EM et al (2012) Comparison between quantitative assessment of bowel wall vascularization by contrast-enhanced ultrasound and results of histopathological scoring in ulcerative colitis. Int J Colorectal Dis 27(2):193–198

26. Deepak P, Bruining DH (2014) Radiographical evaluation of ulcerative colitis. Gastroenterol Rep (Oxf) 2(3):169–177

27. Neri E, Halligan S, Hellström M et al; ESGAR CT Colonography Working Group (2013) The second ESGAR consensus statement on CT colonography. Eur Radiol 23(3):720–729

28. Moulin V, Dellon P, Laurent O et al (2011) Toxic megacolon in patients with severe acute colitis: computed tomographic features. Clin Imaging 35(6):431–436

29. Imbriaco M, Balthazar EJ (2001) Toxic megacolon: role of CT in evaluation and detection of complications. Clin Imaging 25(5):349–354

30. Baumgart DC (ed) (2017) Crohn's disease and ulcerative colitis. From epidemiology and immunobiology to a rational diagnostic and therapeutic approach. Springer, Switzerland
31. Krestin GP, Beyer D, Steinbrich W (1986) Computed tomography in the differential diagnosis of the enlarged retrorectal space. Gastrointest Radiol 11(4):364–369
32. Gore RM (1992) Colonic contour changes in chronic ulcerative colitis: reappraisal of some old concepts. AJR Am J Roentgenol 158(1):59–61
33. Laghi A, Rengo M, Graser A, Iafrate F (2013) Current status on performance of CT colonography and clinical indications. Eur J Radiol 82(8):1192–1200
34. Kirsner JB (ed) (2000) Inflammatory bowel disease. WB Saunders Company, Philadelphia London Toronto Sydney
35. Johnson KT, Hara AK, Johnson CD (2009) Evaluation of colitis: usefulness of CT enterography technique. Emerg Radiol 16(4):277–282
36. Fletcher JC, Fidler JL, Bruining DH, Huprich JE (2011) New concepts in intestinal imaging for inflammatory bowel diseases. Gastroenterology 140(6):1795–1806
37. Yarur AJ, Mandalia AB, Dauer RM et al (2014) Predictive factors for clinically actionable computed tomography findings in inflammatory bowel disease patients seen in the emergency department with acute gastrointestinal symptoms. J Crohns Colitis 8(6):504–512
38. Horsthuis K, Bipat S, Bennink RJ, Stoker J (2008) Inflammatory bowel disease diagnosed with US, MR, scintigraphy, and CT: meta-analysis of prospective studies. Radiology 247(1):64–79
39. Panes J, Jairath V, Levesque BG (2017) Advances in use of endoscopy, radiology, and biomarkers to monitor inflammatory bowel diseases. Gastroenterology 152(2):362–373
40. Maccioni F, Colaiacomo MC, Parlanti S (2005) Ulcerative colitis: value of MR imaging. Abdom Imaging 30(5):584–592
41. Oussalah A, Laurent V, Bruot O et al (2010) Diffusion-weighted magnetic resonance without bowel preparation for detecting colonic inflammation in inflammatory bowel disease. Gut 59(8):1056–1065
42. Ordás I, Rimola J, García-Bosch O et al (2013) Diagnostic accuracy of magnetic resonance colonography for the evaluation of disease activity and severity in ulcerative colitis: a prospective study. Gut 62(11):1566–1572
43. Panes J, Bouzas R, Chaparro M et al (2011) Systematic review: the use of ultrasonography, computed tomography and magnetic resonance imaging for the diagnosis, assessment of activity and abdominal complications of Crohn's disease. Aliment Pharmacol Ther 34(2):125–145
44. Rimola J, Ordás I (2014) MR colonography in inflammatory bowel disease. Magn Reson Imaging Clin N Am 22(1):23–33
45. Schreyer AG, Gölder S, Scheibl K et al (2005) Dark lumen magnetic resonance enteroclysis in combination with MRI colonography for whole bowel assessment in patients with Crohn's disease: first clinical experience. Inflamm Bowel Dis 11(4):388–394
46. Ajaj WM, Lauenstein TC, Pelster G et al (2005) Magnetic resonance colonography for the detection of inflammatory diseases of the large bowel: quantifying the inflammatory activity. Gut 54(2):257–263
47. Langhorst J, Kühle CA, Ajaj W et al (2007) MR colonography without bowel purgation for the assessment of inflammatory bowel diseases: diagnostic accuracy and patient acceptance. Inflamm Bowel Dis 13(8):1001–1008
48. Paolantonio P, Ferrari R, Vecchietti F et al (2009) Current status of MR imaging in the evaluation of IBD in a pediatric population of patients. Eur J Radiol 69(3):418–424
49. Horsthuis K, de Ridder L, Smets AM et al (2010) Magnetic resonance enterography for suspected inflammatory bowel disease in a pediatric population. J Pediatr Gastroenterol Nutr 51(5):603–609

Diagnosis of Ulcerative Colitis: the Role of Endoscopy

4

Gilberto Poggioli, Massimo P. Di Simone, and Laura Vittori

4.1   Introduction

Endoscopy is essential for the diagnosis of ulcerative colitis (UC), the assessment of the extent and severity of the disease, monitoring the response to therapy, and surveillance for dysplasia and cancer [1–3]. In addition, it is fundamental for the postoperative follow-up and the application of therapeutic interventions in case of surgical complications [4, 5].

4.2   Diagnosis

4.2.1   Endoscopic Features of Ulcerative Colitis

Ileocolonoscopy is preferred over sigmoidoscopy for the diagnosis and evaluation of inflammation. It allows direct visualization and biopsy of the mucosa of the rectum, colon, and terminal ileum, and must be performed before initiating any medical treatment. In patients with acute severe colitis who are on corticosteroids, a flexible sigmoidoscopy is suggested in order to avoid complications [3, 5].

In UC, endoscopic changes characteristically start proximal to the ano-rectal junction and extend proximally in a continuous, confluent and concentric fashion. The endoscopic changes may be confined to the rectum (proctitis), affect the left side of the colon (distal or left-sided colitis) or extend beyond the splenic flexure to affect the transverse colon or the cecum and the ascending

M.P. Di Simone (✉)
Department of Medical and Surgical Sciences, University of Bologna, S. Orsola-Malpighi Hospital
Bologna, Italy
e-mail: massimo.disimone@unibo.it

G. Poggioli (Ed), *Ulcerative Colitis*,
Updates in Surgery
DOI: 10.1007/978-88-470-3977-3_4, © Springer-Verlag Italia 2019

colon as well (pancolitis). The demarcation between the inflamed and the normal areas is usually clear and may occur abruptly, especially in distal disease [1, 2].

The early mucosal changes observed are erythema, vascular congestion and loss of vascular pattern. The mucosa is friable with minimal trauma from the endoscope. As inflammation progresses, small ulcers develop and gradually coalesce to form larger ulcers. In this phase, profuse bleeding, and copious exudates are present while, in long-standing disease, mucosal bridge or polyp-like lesions (called pseudopolyps or inflammatory polyps) are frequent. During remission, the mucosa may appear normal but, in patients who have had recurrent attacks, the colon appears to have luminal narrowing with loss of the haustral folds, and atrophy of the mucosa [1, 3, 5].

4.2.2   Discontinuous Inflammation in Ulcerative Colitis

- *Rectal sparing and cecal patch*. Rectal sparing or patchy involvement can be observed in adults who have received prior local or systemic therapy. In particular, rectal sparing occurs if the patient has utilized topical enemas; in children, macroscopic and microscopic rectal sparing has been described prior to treatment. Patchy inflammation in the cecum referred to as a "cecal patch" is observed in patients with left-sided colitis. When there is macroscopic and histological rectal sparing or the presence of a cecal patch in newly diagnosed colitis, evaluation of the small bowel in addition to an ileocolonoscopy is indicated in order to differentiate UC from Crohn's disease (CD) [3, 5].
- *Appendiceal skip lesions*. Appendiceal skip lesions are reported in up to 75% of patients with UC. They have been associated with a better response to medical therapy but a higher risk of pouchitis after ileal pouch anastomosis [3].
- *Backwash ileitis*. Continuous extension of macroscopic or histological inflammation from the cecum into the most distal ileum is observed in up to 20% of patients with pancolitis and is associated with a more refractory course of disease [3].

4.2.3   Mucosal Biopsies

During the procedure, multiple biopsies are necessary for diagnosing UC and excluding other causes of colitis. Following the last ECCO (European Crohn's and Colitis Organisation) guidelines, multiple biopsies from six segments (the terminal ileum, the ascending, transverse, descending and sigmoid colon and the rectum) should be obtained. Multiple biopsies imply a minimum of two representative samples from each segment including macroscopically normal segments [3, 5].

4.2.4   Differential Diagnosis

- *Crohn's disease*. Differentiation between CD and UC has important ramifications for medical therapy, surgical planning, cancer surveillance, and prognosis. None of the endoscopic features are specific for UC or CD in the absence of extracolonic disease. The presence of deep, stellate, linear or serpiginous ulcers, multiple aphthous ulcers and cobblestoning of the mucosa, may suggest a diagnosis of Crohn's colitis over that of UC, in particular if endoscopic findings are defined as "skip lesions" of macroscopically and microscopically uninvolved mucosa. In addition, the presence of ileitis, perianal disease, or visible fistulous opening is indicative of CD [1, 3].
- *Ischemic colitis*. It is usually segmental and tends to affect the splenic flexure and descending colon area, with a normal rectum. There is a sharp transition between the ischemic mucosa and the normal colonic mucosa. Endoscopic findings are: petechial hemorrhages, longitudinal ulcerations, edema and bluish-black blebs [1, 3].
- *Segmental colitis associated with diverticulosis (SCAD)*. SCAD has become increasingly recognized as a distinct clinical and pathological disorder. The inflammatory process involves only the sigmoid colon, often presenting with rectal bleeding. In recent studies, the incidence of SCAD ranged from 0.3% to 2% [3].
- *Radiation proctitis*. Sometimes it can be confused with UC. However, a history of prior radiation for prostatic or uterine cancer, even if temporally distant, can help in the diagnosis [1, 3].
- *Drug-induced colitis*. Non-steroidal anti-inflammatory drugs (NSAIDs), gold, methyldopa and penicillamine can occasionally cause diffuse mild colitis [1, 3].
- *Infective colitis*. A third of the patients presenting with mucoid bloody diarrhea and suspected inflammatory bowel disease (IBD) have an infective etiology. To complicate matters, patients with IBD have the propensity for bacterial superinfection. Endoscopic features favoring infection include yellow tenacious exudates, luminal mucous and an intensely erythematous mucosa. Some infectious diseases – such as *Salmonella* spp., *Shigella* spp. or *Campylobacter* spp. – have endoscopic features similar to UC, while other infections – such as *Yersinia* spp. or cytomegalovirus (CMV) enterocolitis – resemble CD. In the majority of cases, history, presentation, serological tests and stool cultures help in differentiating between infectious colitis and IBD [1, 3]. Infections superimposed on IBD, due to *Clostridium difficile* or CMV, can make the situation more complicated in some instances. While there are no reliable specific features, some clues on endoscopic appearance may point towards non-IBD infective colitis, pending appropriate microbiological testing [3].

4.2.5   Endoscopic Classification of the Disease (Extent and Severity)

A classification according to the extent of the disease is recommended for UC patients. The extent of the disease influences the treatment modality (oral and/ or topical therapy) and prognosis, due to the association between extensive UC and colectomy. Moreover, it is important in determining the beginning and the frequency of surveillance for cancer risk [2, 6].

The Montreal classification of disease extension [7] is commonly used:

E1 = proctitis (the proximal extent of inflammation is distal to the rectosigmoid junction);

E2 = left-sided colitis (inflammation up to the splenic flexure, distal colitis)

E3 = extensive colitis (inflammation proximal to the splenic flexure, pancolitis).

4.2.6   Ulcerative Colitis Scoring Systems

Disease activity in UC has been extensively evaluated using various tools, incorporating both clinical and endoscopic features. These scoring systems have been developed in an attempt to systematically evaluate the response to medical treatment. Although several different scoring systems have been available since the 1960s, they are underused in daily practice [2, 8].

In 1964, Baron et al. proposed a simple scoring system for disease severity, based on a 4-point scale (0–3), mainly according to the severity of the mucosal bleeding and not to the presence of ulceration:

(0) normal mucosa;

(1) mild activity, abnormal mucosa but non-hemorrhagic;

(2) moderate activity, mucosal friability, bleeding to light touch of endoscope;

(3) severe activity, spontaneous mucosal bleeding.

At follow-up, a Baron score ≤1 was defined as endoscopic remission. This score has still not been formally validated [9].

The Mayo score is a global clinical score which establishes the gravity of the disease, taking into account four variables: stool frequency, rectal bleeding, the physician's global assessments and endoscopic findings. The endoscopic component, namely the eMayo Score, was developed in 1987 by Schroeder et al [10]. The endoscopic variables considered were: erythema, vascular pattern, friability, erosions, ulcers and bleeding. The degree of inflammation was based on a 4-point scale (0–3):

(0) normal;

(1) erythema (decreased vascular pattern and mild friability);

(2) marked erythema (absent vascular pattern, friability and erosions);

(3) ulceration and spontaneous bleeding.

The eMayo score is easy to calculate and widely used in clinical trials for the evaluation of treatment efficacy in terms of endoscopic remission. Mucosal healing has been defined as a subscore of 0–1 or as a subscore of 0.

Currently, only the Ulcerative Colitis Endoscopic Index of Severity (UCEIS) and the Ulcerative Colitis Colonoscopic Index of Severity (UCCIS) have received formal validation.

The UCEIS is a newer endoscopic scoring system which grades three endoscopic findings on three to four levels: (1) vascular pattern, (2) bleeding, and (3) erosions/ulcers [11, 12]. Mucosal friability was excluded from the index. It assesses the degree of inflammation with a total score of 3 to 11 (or modified: 0–8) points:

1. vascular pattern [normal (1), patchy obliteration (2) or obliterated (3)];
2. bleeding [none (1), mucosal (2), luminal mild (3), luminal moderate or severe (4)];
3. erosions or ulcers [none (1), erosions (2), superficial ulcer (3) or deep ulcer (4)].

It has been shown that the UCEIS is accurate in assessing disease severity because it is associated with the outcome of acute severe UC [13, 14].

The UCCIS is an endoscopic index which assesses endoscopic severity according to four variables: vascular pattern, granularity, friability, and ulceration. The score calculation requires entering the individual grade of each descriptor into the following formula [15]:

UCCIS = 3.1 × vascular pattern (sum of each segment)
+ 3.6 × granularity (sum of each segment)
+ 3.5 × ulceration (sum of each segment)
+ 2.5 × bleeding/friability (sum of each segment).

All these endoscopic scores indicate the severity of inflammation but not the disease extension, which is a critically important prognostic and therapeutic factor. A recent study proposed the Pancolonic Modified Mayo Score (panMayo) which seems to have both these characteristics. It considers the eMayo score of the 5 colorectal segments. When the eMayo score is ≥2, the sum is multiplied by 3 (IC: Inflammatory Constant) with results from 0 to 45 points in order to clearly differentiate the active from the inactive disease. Some authors have demonstrated a correlation between the UCEIS and the Mayo score, and also with clinical and laboratory findings [16, 17].

In patients with ulcerative colitis, a periodic restaging of the disease is recommended, in order to establish disease activity or endoscopic remission. The evidence of "mucosal healing" is a good outcome predictor. The definition of "mucosal healing" can vary from light erythema, granularity and/or friability to more specific definitions: normal mucosa with the absence of all ulceration (both microscopic and macroscopic), giving a sigmoidoscopy score of 0 with no friability. There are no strict recommendations regarding the timing of restaging; it is usually appropriate at relapse, for steroid-dependent or refractory ulcerative colitis or when considering colectomy [2, 5].

4.3   Surveillance

It is generally stated that colorectal cancer (CRC) is strictly linked to UC. Data in the literature have reported an estimate of risk which varied from 0.2% to 2.0% at 10 years of disease up to 3.1% to 18.0% at 30 years [18, 19]. A decreased incidence of CRC has been observed in recent years. A recent study has reported a CRC cumulative incidence of 1% at 10 years, 3% at 20 years and 7% at 30 years. This could also be due to an improvement in screening and surveillance strategies, the introduction of drugs which control inflammation more effectively, or the changing approach to maintenance therapy or colectomy [20, 21].

The risk of colorectal cancer in ulcerative colitis depends on the duration of the disease, the extent of the colitis, and severe or persistent activity. The occurrence of cancer increased indicatively after 8–10 years of disease duration, particularly in patients with extensive colitis [22–24]. Primary sclerosing cholangitis (PSC), family history of colorectal cancer and presence of post-inflammatory polyps are considered additional risk factors for CRC [25, 26].

The task of surveillance endoscopy is the early identification of dysplasia or cancer in order to reduce possible morbidity or mortality [3–5]. Screening for CRC is generally recommended in patients with IBD, an ileal pouch-anal anastomosis (IPAA) and in patients with undetermined or unclassified colitis. In UC the first screening endoscopy should be performed 8 years after diagnosis, but stratifying patients according to their individual risk factors is recommended. Patients with high risk factors, such as concomitant PSC, previous detection of dysplasia, extensive colitis, and presence of active severe inflammation or stricture, should undergo surveillance endoscopy after one year. In particular, when there is a diagnosis of PSC annual endoscopy is recommended. Intermediate risk factors, such as left-sided colitis, mild or moderate active inflammation, post-inflammatory polyps or first-degree relatives with CRC who are under 50 years of age, should be evaluated every 2 or 3 years. Patients who are at low or no risk should undergo endoscopic surveillance every 5 years [27–29]. Endoscopic surveillance should also be carried out during remission of disease and a good quality of preparation is recommended.

The techniques of choice are chromoendoscopy using methylene blue or indigo carmine, taking targeted biopsies, or white light endoscopy with random quadrantic biopsies every 10 cm. [30, 31]. New advanced imaging techniques (magnification endoscopy, dye-based and dye-less chromoendoscopy, endomicroscopy and endocytoscopy) are under study for the assessment of mucosal inflammation and dysplasia development in IBD; however, current data do not support their routine use [32–34]. Subramanian et al., showed the usefulness of high-definition colonoscopy in dysplasia detection during surveillance in pa-

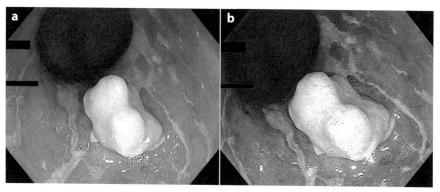

Fig. 4.1 Inflammatory polyp of the rectum in long standing ulcerative colitis visualized by high-definition standard white-light endoscopy (**a**) and by high-definition narrow-banding imaging (**b**)

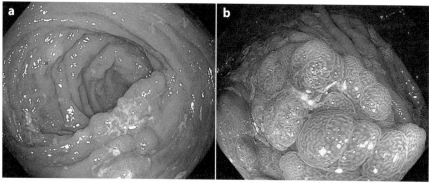

Fig. 4.2 View of a large sessile polypoid lesion (Paris type Is) of the hepatic flexure of the colon using high-definition white-light endoscopy (**a**) and narrow-banding imaging (**b**). Histopathological analysis revealed low-grade dysplasia

tients with IBD [35]. However, in a recent meta-analysis, chromoendoscopy was still superior to white light endoscopy for the detection of dysplasia in IBD, even with high-definition endoscopy. While no difference could be demonstrated for narrow band imaging (NBI) in comparison with the other two modalities [36]. NBI is an optical chromoendoscopy technology which uses filters to enhance the contrast of the mucosa and the vasculature (Fig. 4.1).

In 2017, the ECCO published guidelines regarding cancer surveillance for colorectal cancer in UC [5]. According to the SCENIC international consensus, terms, such as dysplasia-associated lesions or masses (DALMs), adenoma-like, non-adenoma-like and flat lesions should be discontinued [37]. Using the Paris Classification, dysplasia should be described as polypoid, non-polypoid or macroscopically invisible (Fig. 4.2). Irrespective of the degree of dysplasia, visible well-defined polyps should be endoscopically excised and biopsies of the adjacent mucosa should be taken [5]. In the absence of both dysplasia in the adjacent mucosa and synchronous dysplasia, continued surveillance is recommended. Since the risk of developing additional dysplasia in patients presenting this scenario is increased 10-fold, close endoscopic follow-up (after 3–6 months) is required [38]. In the case of dysplasia in the adjacent mucosa or synchronous dysplasia, a total colectomy is advised.

Conversely, a surgical approach with total colectomy is strongly recommended in patients with non-polypoid dysplasia due to its elevated correlation with metachronous or synchronous CRC and to its multifocal location [39]. The true risk of invisible dysplasia, detected by random biopsies, is very difficult to estimate. For this reason, a repeated endoscopy in a reference center for IBD is recommended. If the second endoscopy confirms the presence of non-visible dysplasia, the patient should be managed in relation to the degree of dysplasia. In particular, a diagnosis of high-grade dysplasia requires a surgical approach with total colectomy [40].

In younger patients with typical postsurgical quality of life, colectomy for invisible low-grade dysplasia may be more effective clinically and more cost-effective than surveillance [41]. Recently, a Dutch study investigated the long-term risk of advanced neoplasia after colonic low-grade dysplasia in a nationwide cohort of IBD patients [42]. The cumulative incidence of advanced neoplasia was 21.9% and 29.9% after 15 and 20 years, respectively. Therefore, advising a colectomy is also correct in the case of low-grade dysplasia. If the patient refuses surgery, a repeat endoscopy with additional random biopsies is recommended within 3 months and then annual surveillance should be carried out [3].

Accurate surveillance is important in order to guarantee a better life expectancy for the patient [43].

4.4   Post-surgical Evaluation

4.4.1   Ileal Pouch Endoscopy

Ileal pouch-anal anastomosis has become the surgical treatment of choice for restoration of bowel continuity after colectomy and has been associated with acceptable bowel function. Endoscopy plays an important role in postoperative monitoring of disease status [5, 44, 45].

It must examine all segments of the IPAA (the anastomosis, the cuff, the pouch body, the tip of the J, the afferent limb and the loop ileostomy closure site). In the 3-stage procedure, pouchoscopy is suggested between the 2nd and the 3rd stages, in order to confirm the normal healing of the pouch and the pouch-anal sutures before the ileostomy closure. Usually this procedure is performed 2 months after the proctectomy and the construction. An endoscopic follow-up is useful after ileostomy closure for monitoring pouch functioning and the mucosal conditions of the pouch, and for diagnosing complications. If complications occur, endoscopic therapy can be carried out and it has been shown to be safe and effective, allowing a majority of patients to retain their pouches [46].

4.4.2   Surgery-associated Complications

The most common causes of pouch failure are pouch leaks and strictures; other complications are bleeding, and ischemia.

4.4.2.1   Pouch Leaks

Pouch leaks occur early after IPAA; the most common locations are the pouch-anal anastomosis and the tip of the "J" [44].

Anastomotic leakage occurs in 4% of IPAA patients in the presence of a protective stoma, and in up to 15% in the non-diverted pouches. It may be associated with a posterior presacral cavity or, in women with an anterior pouch-vaginal fistula. In the presence of fistulous complication, other causes of this manifestation must be excluded, such as ischemic damage, cryptoglandular abscess formation and undiagnosed CD [4, 5]. A careful pouchoscopy can show the defect of the circular pouch-anal anastomosis; however, to clearly delineate the fistula tract and depth, the presacral cavity, and to determine the direction of treatment, a contrasted pouchogram and pelvic magnetic resonance imaging are needed [44].

Endoscopy can be used in treating drainage of the collection, which may be adjacent to the leakage, and for the closure of the fistula using the clipping system or Endo-Sponge vacuum assisted drainage (B. Braun Medical B.V., Melsungen, Germany), specifically designed for small leaks. In 2008, Weidenhagen described a novel approach for treating anastomotic leakage and presacral abscess after resection of the rectum, using the Endo-Sponge [47]. It is an open-pored polyurethane sponge (connected to a vacuum suction bottle in order to create constant negative pressure) which is endoscopically placed in the presacral cavity. By changing the Endo-Sponge twice a week and tapering the size of the sponge systematically, the abscess cavity gradually collapses. Based on this experience, Gardenbroek et al. have proposed treating anastomotic leakage after IPAA with early surgical closure of the cavity after a short period of Endo-Sponge [48]. Closure of the anastomotic defect was achieved in all patients (n=15) after a median of 48 (25–103) days as compared with 52% (n=16) in the conventional treatment group (loop ileostomy and occasional drainage of the presacral cavity).

This system has recently been introduced and studied at our institution. The vacuum-assisted closure therapy was utilized in 8 patients as a unique treatment

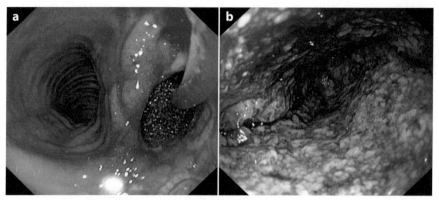

Fig. 4.3 Pouch-anal anastomotic leak. The Endo-Sponge device is inserted in the anastomotic gap
(**a**). After removing the sponge, the cavity appears clean and covered by granulation tissue (**b**)

for anastomotic leaks following IPAA (Fig. 4.3). The complete healing of the
leak was documented in all patients after a median of 60 (24–90) days from the
first treatment [49].

For the management of leaking at the tip of the "J" pouch, Kochhar and
Shen, have proposed using the OTSC system (Over-The-Scope Clipping, Ovesco
Endoscopy USA, Cary, NC), a new type of endoscopic clip, having a particular
design and used to treat non-variceal gastrointestinal bleeding, fistula of the
gastrointestinal tract, and esophageal perforation. Of the 12 patients presented
in this case series, 8 (66.6%) were successfully treated with OTSC, obviating
surgical repair [50].

4.4.2.2 Pouch Sinus

Pouch sinus is typically a later presentation of an initial anastomotic leak. The
most common location of a pouch sinus is the pouch-anal anastomotic site,
which is frequently located at the presacral space.

Endoscopic treatment usually includes periodic incision and drainage of
the chronically infected superficial sinuses to promote secondary healing and
closure [44]. However, this conservative treatment may take up to 12 months
before these sinuses heal. In some cases, fibrin glue injection of the sinus may
be attempted to shorten the healing time [51].

Moreover, the use of endoscopic needle knife therapy for the treatment of
simple, shallow (<5 cm in depth) presacral sinus has recently been proposed.
In one experience, the procedure was performed in 65 patients with or without
a protecting diverting ileostomy; 84.6% of patients with a simple, short sinus,
achieved a complete or partial response [52, 53].

Pouch-vaginal fistula (PVF) in IPAA is a major source of discomfort for the
patient, increases morbidity and is a cause of pouch failure. A diagnosis of PVF

is mainly based on symptoms, but endoscopic and radiographic documentation is often needed for the differential diagnosis and the choice of treatment [54, 55].

4.4.2.3 Pouch Strictures

Pouch strictures are one of the most frequent adverse events after IPAA, with a reported frequency ranging from 10% to 17% [44]. Common locations are at the anastomosis, pouch body, afferent limb and the site of prior ileostomy. It is important to differentiate between iatrogenic strictures and misdiagnosed CD. In CD, stenosis does not usually involve anastomosis or other sutures, and disease characteristics are present (such as segmental ulcers, nodularity, exudate).

The majority of anastomotic strictures are self-limiting web-type strictures which are successfully treated with digital dilatation, or with corticosteroid injections or bougie dilations [56–60].

Long, fibrotic strictures refractory to pneumatic dilations may be treated with endoscopic therapy. Endoscopic needle knife stricturotomy (NKSt) was carried out in 85 IBD patients with primary or secondary stenosis. Only 13 patients (15.3%) required surgery, and, of a total of 272 NKSt procedures performed, only 10 adverse events (3.7%) occurred (9 bleeding events and 1 perforation) [61].

4.4.3   Inflammatory Complications

Inflammatory long-term adverse events of IPAA include pouchitis, "cuffitis", pre-pouch ileitis, irritable pouch syndrome and CD of the pouch, with a reported pouch failure incidence of 3.5% to 15% [4, 5, 62, 63].

4.4.3.1 Pouchitis

Pouchitis is the most common long-term adverse event after the procedure.

Endoscopic findings consistent with pouchitis include erythema, edema, granularity, friability, spontaneous or contact bleeding, erosions and ulcerations [5]. Pouchitis is not a homogenous disease entity. In primary or idiopathic pouchitis the etiopathogenesis is still unclear (dysbiosis and altered mucosal immune response), while in secondary pouchitis a specific cause is known: infection (i.e., *C. difficile*, CMV), ischemic, non-steroidal anti-inflammatory drug-induced, autoimmune-associated infection or CD. In particular, ischemic pouchitis may be related to the surgical construction of the pouch, including disruption of the vessels supplying the distal ileum or the tension of the mesentery during the IPAA construction. Mucosal lesions are often asymmetric (i.e., only the afferent limb, the pouch body or the distal pouch body/suture line is involved) [64]. Endoscopic and histologic assessment facilitates the diagnosis of pouchitis and/or the exclusion of other causes of the symptoms.

Two scoring systems (combining clinical symptoms, endoscopic findings, and histologic feature) have been developed to diagnose pouchitis and to assess disease severity: the pouchitis disease activity index and the pouchitis activity score [65, 66].

4.4.3.2 Cuffitis

Cuffitis refers to inflammation of the rectal cuff and is common in IPAA constructed with stapled anastomosis without mucosectomy. With this technique, a 1–2 cm ring of rectal mucosa remains between the anastomosis and the dentate line; there is a high risk of inflammation and the necessity of surveillance for dysplasia [5].

4.4.3.3 Pre-pouch Ileitis

This is not a well-known complication of surgically treated UC and can involve acute or chronic inflammation of the afferent limb of the pouch. Pouchoscopy shows a friable granular mucosa with ulcers and, in 50% of patients, a stricture which requires dilatation is present [67].

4.4.4   Neoplastic Complications

In a meta-analysis of published studies, the prevalence and incidence of CRC after colectomy was less than 3%; in patients receiving IPAA it was less than 1% [68]. In a recent study the long-term risk of cancer in a national cohort of patients with UC and IPAA was very rare 0.12% [69].

References

1. Panagiotakopoulos D, Panos M (2006) Endoscopy in inflammatory bowel disease. Ann Gastroenterol 19(1):42–54
2. Dignass A, Eliakim R, Magro F et al (2012) Second European evidence-based consensus on the diagnosis and management of ulcerative colitis part 1: definitions and diagnosis. J Crohns Colitis 2012 6(10):965–990
3. Annese V, Daperno M, Rutter MD et al; European Crohn's and Colitis Organisation (2013) European evidence-based consensus for endoscopy in inflammatory bowel disease. J Crohns Colitis 7(12):982–1018
4. American Society for Gastrointestinal Endoscopy Standards of Practice Committee, Shergill AK, Lightdale JR, Bruining DH et al (2015) The role of endoscopy in inflammatory bowel disease. Gastrointest Endosc 81(5):1101–1121
5. Magro F, Gionchetti G, Eliakim R et al; European Crohn's and Colitis Organisation [ECCO] (2017) Third European evidence-based consensus on diagnosis and management of ulcerative colitis. Part 1: definitions, diagnosis, extra-intestinal manifestations, pregnancy, cancer surveillance, surgery, and ileo-anal pouch disorders. J Crohns Colitis 11(6):649–670

6. D'Haens G, Sandborn WJ, Feagan BG et al (2007) A review of activity indices and efficacy end points for clinical trials of medical therapy in adults with ulcerative colitis. Gastroenterology 132(2):763–786

7. Satsangi J, Silverberg MS, Vermeire S, Colombel JF (2006) The Montreal classification of inflammatory bowel disease: controversies, consensus, and implications. Gut 55(6):749–753

8. Mohammed Vashist N, Samaan M, Mosli MH et al (2018) Endoscopic scoring indices for evaluation of disease activity in ulcerative colitis. Cochrane Database Syst Rev 2009(1): CD011450

9. Baron JH, Connell AM, Lennard-Jones JE (1964) Variation between observers in describing mucosal appearances in proctocolitis. Br Med J 1(5375):89–92

10. Schroeder KW, Tremaine WJ, Ilstrup DM (1987) Coated oral 5-aminosalicylic acid therapy for mildly to moderately active ulcerative colitis. A randomized study. N Engl J Med 317(26):1625–1629

11. Travis SP, Schnell D, Krzeski P et al (2012) Developing an instrument to assess the endoscopic severity of ulcerative colitis: the Ulcerative Colitis Endoscopic Index of Severity (UCEIS). Gut 61(4):535–542

12. Travis SP, Schnell D, Feagan BG et al (2015) The impact of clinical information on the assessment of endoscopic activity: characteristics of the Ulcerative Colitis Endoscopic Index of Severity [UCEIS]. J Crohns Colitis 9(8):607–616

13. Ikeya K, Hanai H, Sugimoto K et al (2016) The Ulcerative Colitis Endoscopic Index of Severity more accurately reflects clinical outcomes and long-term prognosis than the Mayo Endoscopic Score. J Crohns Colitis 10(3):286–295

14. Arai M, Naganuma M, Sugimoto S et al (2016) The Ulcerative Colitis Endoscopic Index of Severity is useful to predict medium-to-long-term prognosis in ulcerative colitis patients with clinical remission. J Crohns Colitis 10(11):1303–1309

15. Samuel S, Bruining DH, Loftus EV Jr et al (2013) Validation of the Ulcerative Colitis Colonoscopic Index of Severity and its correlation with disease activity measures. Clin Gastroenterol Hepatol 11(1):49–54

16. Lobatón T, Bessissow T, De Hertogh G et al (2015) The Modified Mayo Endoscopic Score (MMES): a new index for the assessment of extension and severity of endoscopic activity in ulcerative colitis patients. J Crohns Colitis 9(10):846–852

17. Bálint A, Farkas K, Szepes Z et al (2018) How disease extent can be included in the endoscopic activity index of ulcerative colitis: the panMayo score, a promising scoring system. BMC Gastroenterol 18(1):7

18. Eaden JA, Abrams KR, Mayberry JF (2001) The risk of colorectal cancer in ulcerative colitis: a meta-analysis. Gut 48(4):526–535

19. Kiran RP, Khoury W, Church JM et al (2010) Colorectal cancer complicating inflammatory bowel disease: similarities and differences between Crohn's and ulcerative colitis based on three decades of experience. Ann Surg 252(2):330–335

20. Jess T, Horváth-Puhó E, Fallingborg J et al (2013) Cancer risk in inflammatory bowel disease according to patient phenotype and treatment: a Danish population-based cohort study. Am J Gastroenterol 108(12):1869–1876

21. Choi CH, Rutter MD, Askari A et al (2015) Forty-year analysis of colonoscopic surveillance program for neoplasia in ulcerative colitis: an updated overview. Am J Gastroenterol 110(7):1022–1034

22. Winther KV, Jess T, Langholz E et al (2004) Long-term risk of cancer in ulcerative colitis: a population-based cohort study from Copenhagen County. Clin Gastroenterol Hepatol 2(12):1088–1095

23. Lutgens MW, Vleggaar FP, Schipper ME et al (2008) High frequency of early colorectal cancer in inflammatory bowel disease. Gut 57(9):1246–1251

24. Beaugerie L, Svrcek M, Seksik P et al; CESAME Study Group (2013) Risk of colorectal high-grade dysplasia and cancer in a prospective observational cohort of patients with inflammatory bowel disease. Gastroenterology 145(1):166–175

25. Bergeron V, Vienne A, Sokol H et al (2010) Risk factors for neoplasia in inflammatory bowel disease patients with pancolitis. Am J Gastroenterol 105(11):2405–2411

26. Jørgensen KK, Lindström L, Cvancarova M et al (2012) Colorectal neoplasia in patients with primary sclerosing cholangitis undergoing liver transplantation: a Nordic multicenter study. Scand J Gastroenterol 47(8–9):1021–1029

27. Befrits R, Ljung T, Jaramillo E, Rubio C (2002) Low-grade dysplasia in extensive, long-standing inflammatory bowel disease: a follow-up study. Dis Colon Rectum 45(5):615–620

28. Soetikno RM, Lin OS, Heidenreich PA et al (2002) Increased risk of colorectal neoplasia in patients with primary sclerosing cholangitis and ulcerative colitis: a meta-analysis. Gastrointest Endosc 56(1):48–54

29. Jess T, Loftus EV Jr, Velayos FS et al (2006) Incidence and prognosis of colorectal dysplasia in inflammatory bowel disease: a population-based study from Olmsted County, Minnesota. Inflamm Bowel Dis 12(8):669–676

30. Hlavaty T, Huorka M, Koller T et al (2011) Colorectal cancer screening in patients with ulcerative and Crohn's colitis with use of colonoscopy, chromoendoscopy and confocal endomicroscopy. Eur J Gastroenterol Hepatol 23(8):680–689

31. Watanabe T, Ajioka Y, Mitsuyama K et al (2016) Comparison of targeted vs random biopsies for surveillance of ulcerative colitis-associated colorectal cancer. Gastroenterology 151(6):1122–1130

32. Bojarski C (2009) Malignant transformation in inflammatory bowel disease: prevention, surveillance and treatment – new techniques in endoscopy. Dig Dis 27(4):571–575

33. Goetz M (2011) Colonoscopic surveillance in inflammatory bowel disease: state of the art reduction of biopsies. Dig Dis 29(Suppl 1):36–40

34. Rath T, Tontini GE, Neurath MF, Neumann H (2015) From the surface to the single cell: novel endoscopic approaches in inflammatory bowel disease. World J Gastroenterol 21(40):11260–11272

35. Subramanian V, Ramappa V, Telakis E et al (2013) Comparison of high definition with standard white light endoscopy for detection of dysplastic lesions during surveillance colonoscopy in patients with colonic inflammatory bowel disease. Inflamm Bowel Dis 19(2):350–355

36. Har-Noy O, Katz L, Avni T et al (2017) Chromoendoscopy, narrow-band imaging or white light endoscopy for neoplasia detection in inflammatory bowel diseases. Dig Dis Sci 62(11):2982–2990

37. Laine L, Kaltenbach T, Barkun A et al; SCENIC Guideline Development Panel (2015) SCENIC international consensus statement on surveillance and management of dysplasia in inflammatory bowel disease. Gastroenterology 148(3):639–651

38. Wanders LK, Dekker E, Pullens B et al (2014) Cancer risk after resection of polypoid dysplasia in patients with longstanding ulcerative colitis: a meta-analysis. Clin Gastroenterol Hepatol 12(5):756–764

39. Choi CH, Ignjatovic-Wilson A, Askari A et al (2015) Low-grade dysplasia in ulcerative colitis: risk factors for developing high-grade dysplasia or colorectal cancer. Am J Gastroenterol 110(10):1461–1467

40. Van Assche G, Dignass A, Bokemeyer B et al; European Crohn's and Colitis Organisation (2013) Second European evidence-based consensus on the diagnosis and management of ulcerative colitis part 3: special situations. J Crohns Colitis 7(1):1–33

41. Parker B, Buchanan J, Wordsworth S et al (2017) Surgery versus surveillance in ulcerative colitis patients with endoscopically invisible low-grade dysplasia: a cost-effectiveness analysis. Gastrointest Endosc 86(6):1088–1099

42. de Jong M, van Tilburg S, Nissen L et al (2018) OP036 Long-term risk of advanced neoplasia after colonic low-grade dysplasia in patients with inflammatory bowel disease: a nationwide cohort study. J Crohn Colitis 12 (Suppl 1):S026

43. Cole EB, Shah Y, McLean LP et al (2018) Frequency of surveillance and impact of surveillance colonoscopies in patients with ulcerative colitis who developed colorectal cancer. Clin Colorectal Cancer 17(2):e289–e292

44. Shen B (2010) Diagnosis and management of postoperative ileal pouch disorders. Clin Colon Rectal Surg 23(4):259–268
45. Shen B (2016) The evaluation of postoperative patients with ulcerative colitis. Gastrointest Endosc Clin N Am 26(4):669–677
46. Modha K, Navaneethan U (2014) Advanced therapeutic endoscopist and inflammatory bowel disease: dawn of a new role. World J Gastroenterol 20(13):3485–3494
47. Weidenhagen R, Gruetzner KU, Wiecken T et al (2008) Endoscopic vacuum-assisted closure of anastomotic leakage following anterior resection of the rectum: a new method. Surg Endosc 22(8):1818–1825
48. Gardenbroek TJ, Musters GD, Buskens CJ et al (2015) Early reconstruction of the leaking ileal pouch-anal anastomosis: a novel solution to an old problem. Colorectal Dis 17(5):426–432
49. Rottoli M, Di Simone MP, Vallicelli C et al (2018) Endoluminal vacuum-assisted therapy as treatment for anastomotic leak after ileal pouch-anal anastomosis: a pilot study. Tech Coloproctol 22(3):223–229
50. Kochhar GS, Shen B (2017) Endoscopic treatment of leak at the tip of the "J" ileal pouch. Endosc Int Open 5(1):E64–E66
51. Swain BT, Ellis CN (2004) Fibrin glue treatment of low rectal and pouch-anal anastomotic sinuses. Dis Colon Rectum 47(2):253–255
52. Lian L, Geisler D, Shen B (2010) Endoscopic needle knife treatment of chronic presacral sinus at the anastomosis at an ileal pouch-anal anastomosis. Endoscopy 42(Suppl 2):E14
53. Wu XR, Wong RC, Shen B (2013) Endoscopic needle-knife therapy for ileal pouch sinus: a novel approach for the surgical adverse event (with video). Gastrointest Endosc 78(6):875–885
54. Shah NS, Remzi F, Massmann A et al (2003) Management and treatment outcome of pouch-vaginal fistulas following restorative proctocolectomy. Dis Colon Rectum 46(7):911–917
55. Mallick IH, Hull TL, Remzi FH, Kiran RP (2014) Management and outcome of pouch-vaginal fistulas after IPAA surgery. Dis Colon Rectum 57(4):490–496
56. Shen B, Lian L, Kiran RP et al (2011) Efficacy and safety of endoscopic treatment of ileal pouch strictures. Inflamm Bowel Dis 17(12):2527–2535
57. Bharadwaj S, Shen B (2017) Medical, endoscopic, and surgical management of ileal pouch strictures (with video). Gastrointest Endosc 86(1):59–73
58. Prudhomme M, Dozois RR, Godlewski G et al (2003) Anal canal strictures after ileal pouch-anal anastomosis. Dis Colon Rectum 46(1):20–23
59. Shen B, Fazio VW, Remzi FH et al (2004) Endoscopic balloon dilation of ileal pouch strictures. Am J Gastroenterol 99(12):2340–2347
60. Lucha PA Jr, Fticsar JE, Francis MJ (2005) The strictured anastomosis: successful treatment by corticosteroid injections – report of three cases and review of the literature. Dis Colon Rectum 48(4):862–865
61. Lan N, Shen B (2017) Endoscopic stricturotomy with needle knife in the treatment of strictures from inflammatory bowel disease. Inflamm Bowel Dis 23(4):502–513
62. Shen B, Lashner BA (2008) Diagnosis and treatment of pouchitis. Gastroenterol Hepatol (NY) 4(5):355–361
63. Zezos P, Saibil F (2015) Inflammatory pouch disease: the spectrum of pouchitis. World J Gastroenterol 21(29):8739–8752
64. Shen B, Plesec TP, Remer E et al (2010) Asymmetric endoscopic inflammation of the ileal pouch: a sign of ischemic pouchitis? Inflamm Bowel Dis 16(5):836–846
65. Sandborn WJ, Tremaine WJ, Batts KP et al (1994) Pouchitis After Ileal Pouch-Anal Anastomosis: A Pouchitis Disease Activity Index. Mayo Clin Proc 69(5):409–415
66. Heuschen UA, Allemeyer EH, Hinz U et al (2002) Diagnosing pouchitis: comparative validation of two scoring systems in routine follow-up. Dis Colon Rectum 45(6):776–786
67. Rottoli M, Vallicelli C, Bigonzi E et al (2018) Prepouch ileitis after ileal pouch-anal anastomosis: patterns of presentation and risk factors for failure of treatment. J Crohns Colitis12(3):273–279

68. Derikx LAAP, Nissen LHC, Smits LJT et al (2016) Risk of neoplasia after colectomy in patients with inflammatory bowel disease: a systematic review and meta-analysis. Clin Gastroenterol Hepatol 14(6):798–806
69. Mark-Christensen A, Erichsen R, Brandsborg S et al (2018) Long-term risk of cancer following ileal pouch-anal anastomosis for ulcerative colitis. J Crohns Colitis 12(1):57–62

Diagnosis of Ulcerative Colitis: Morphology and Histopathological Characteristics

5

Antonietta D'Errico and Deborah Malvi

5.1 Role of Histology

The role of the pathologist in the clinical management of inflammatory bowel disease (IBD) is to diagnose and define the type of IBD, to define the status of the colonic mucosa (active or chronic), to identify the presence of dysplasia and to exclude complications [1, 2].

Moreover, histology provides information regarding the phase of IBD and mucosal status, unlike that of the endoscopic examination; endoscopic evaluation can be different from histological assessment [3] and endoscopic mucosal healing (MH) does not necessarily correspond to MH at a histological level [4, 5]. For these reasons, guidelines consider histological evaluation to be the gold standard for the management of patients [6].

Several studies have confirmed that histology is a better indicator of the inflammatory status of the colonic mucosa than endoscopy, for the most part in the presence of only minimal or mild mucosal inflammation; Truelove et al. have reported that 40–60% of normal endoscopic examinations of ulcerative colitis (UC) patients had mild to moderate histologically evident mucosal inflammation [7]. Thomas et al. reported only low agreement between clinical status, endoscopy and histology, and the study conducted by Rosenberg et al. showed that more than 50% of patients in clinical remission had histological evidence of inflammation, independent of the therapeutic regimen used [8, 9]. Of interest, in the latter study, islands of activity in the right colon were found during complete endoscopy (i.e., cecal patch) in patients with only distal UC, indicating a key role for a total and complete endoscopic examination with biopsy [9].

A. D'Errico (✉)
Department of Experimental Diagnostic and Specialty Medicine, University of Bologna,
S. Orsola-Malpighi Hospital
Bologna, Italy
e-mail: antonietta.derrico@unibo.it

G. Poggioli (Ed), *Ulcerative Colitis*,
Updates in Surgery
DOI: 10.1007/978-88-470-3977-3_5, © Springer-Verlag Italia 2019

Histologically, the remission of UC is defined by the presence of complete mucosal healing [10, 11] or by the presence of residual features of chronicity [12, 13]. The lymphomonocytic infiltrate of the lamina propria can be increased or decreased, and basal cell plasmacytosis is no longer apparent.

Long-term remission, a long relapse-free period, and reduction in hospitalization and surgical treatment have been proven to be related to MH [14]. Moreover, MH has been associated with a reduction in cancer risk and cancer-related mortality [14], indicating that the persistence of inflammatory activity may play a role in IBD-related carcinogenesis [15, 16].

The presence of basal plasmacytosis in an otherwise remission phase of UC has been associated with a shorter disease-free period [17]. Conversely, the persistence of an increased inflammatory infiltrate of the lamina propria and the presence of other signs of activity are associated with an increased risk of relapse [9, 17–19] and colectomy [20, 21]. In particular, the study of Tanaka et al. has proposed five histological parameters to predict the success or failure of the medical treatment; moreover, it demonstrated that non-responding UC patients had a higher number of eosinophils of the lamina propria, suggesting that they could be a possible sign of the failure of steroid therapy [22–24].

Several studies have analyzed the predictive factors for colectomy in UC patients: Daperno et al. [25] reported the presence of "slow" and "early" steroid responders; Molnár et al. 2011 [26] demonstrated that the colectomy rate was higher in non-responding patients and that approximately 40% of patients had undergone colectomy the following year despite the good response to the second-line rescue therapy.

Among pediatric UC patients, there are some interesting articles correlating the clinical, biological and histological parameters with clinical relapse, starting with the study of Bitton et al. in 2001 [17], in which basal plasmacytosis and rectal biopsies had a significant predictive value.

In spite of the key role of histological evaluation in demonstrating mucosal alterations in UC patients, some limitations remain, mainly due to the use of clinical and endoscopic endpoints in routine clinical practice [27] related to the lack of standard histological reporting and validated histological scoring systems, and especially to the lack of reproducible criteria for defining MH [28].

5.2   Histological Features

Ulcerative colitis is defined as an idiopathic inflammatory process of the large bowel and rectum, and diagnosis is based on medical history, clinical evaluation together with endoscopic and histological confirmation of typical signs, and evaluation of the serological markers [29].

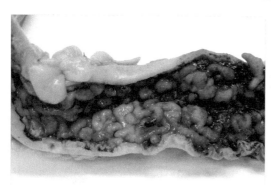

Fig. 5.1 Colectomy specimen, left-sided colon: the typical presentation of ulcerative colitis showing a cobblestone and granular appearance of the mucosa with superficial ulcerations

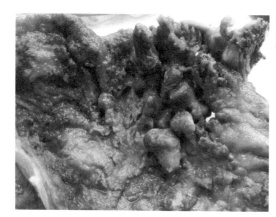

Fig. 5.2 Left-sided colectomy showing pseudopolyps in the context of widespread mucosal ulceration

Macroscopic examination of the resected specimen classically shows the presence of a continuous alteration of the mucosa from the rectum to the proximal colon, with a gradual decrease in the severity of the disease and a sharp demarcation between the uninvolved and the diseased mucosa. The typical presentation of UC consists of a friable and granular appearance of the mucosal surface, with the presence of superficial ulcerations (Fig. 5.1). In the more severe cases, these can undermine the adjacent mucosa and penetrate deep through the muscularis mucosae [30, 31] producing deep fissures and fistulas in cases of fulminant colitis which can give rise to the so-called Crohn-like colitis appearance [32, 33].

The appearance of pseudopolyps (Fig. 5.2) is due to the presence of an island of normal/healed mucosa in the context of extensive ulceration; this presentation is typical in the left colon except for the rectum.

Chronic inactive UC is characterized by the presence of atrophic and flat mucosa with the disappearance of the typical haustration.

The unusual macroscopic presentation of UC shows rectal sparing (especially in adults with fulminant colitis or in patients receiving topical treatments) [32, 34–37], a cecal patch (left-sided colon involvement associated with the presence of active colitis in the cecum, around the appendiceal orifice) [36–40] and backwash ileitis. Backwash ileitis can be found in 20% of patients with diffuse UC without a cecal involvement [41–43]. In a minority of cases, UC can produce strictures due to the presence of marked mucosal and submucosal fibrosis [44].

Histology is a key step in the management of clinical patient care; it is therefore not only used to confirm the endoscopic/clinical suspicion, but it is also helpful in the patient follow-up to determine the grade of inflammatory activity and the grade of MH, thus helping to predict the risk of relapse [4, 17, 45]. For a correct histological interpretation, clinicians should send an adequate number of well-oriented biopsies from at least five sites including the terminal ileum and rectum, each in a separate biopsy-box, and a clinical report including the onset and duration of the disease, the therapy carried out and the status of the patient at the time of the procedure [46].

Studies have demonstrated that histology is a better predictor of MH than endoscopy [47, 48] demonstrating that complete MH during UC is associated with a lower rate of immunosuppressive therapy, lower rates of hospitalization and a lower risk of colectomy and malignancy [21, 49]. Mucosal architecture distortion with gland branching and deformation, and diffuse transmucosal inflammation with basal crypt plasmacytosis are the typical histological features of UC. The presence of an active inflammatory component causing cryptitis and crypt abscesses with mucin depletion [50–52] and gland regeneration defines the active phase of the inflammatory process. Typically, the inflammatory infiltrate is diffuse and continuous [44, 53, 54] without "skip lesions" and with the highest grade of severity in the rectum (Fig. 5.3).

The presence of mucosal atrophy characterizes the quiescent phase of the disease together with Paneth cell metaplasia, inflammatory pseudopolyps and hypertrophy of the muscularis mucosae [55]. Granulomas are not generally considered features diagnostic of UC (Fig. 5.4); they are rarely found related to mucin extravasation in active UC with cryptitis and ruptured glands [56].

The histological spectrum of UC can be very variable, depending not only on the phase of the disease (i.e., chronic active, chronic inactive or simply active colitis) but also on disease duration and the type of treatment received.

At the very beginning of the disease, histology may not show the typically expected alterations since only 20% of patients have crypt distortion. Basal cell plasmacytosis (one of the strongest predictors of IBD together with an increase in lymphocytes and plasma cells, and gland distortion is found in only fewer than 50% of patients and when present, it can be very focal [18]. On the other hand, the diagnosis of long-standing UC, is commonly characterized by architectural gland distortion, mucosal atrophy with a reduction in crypt numbers and an

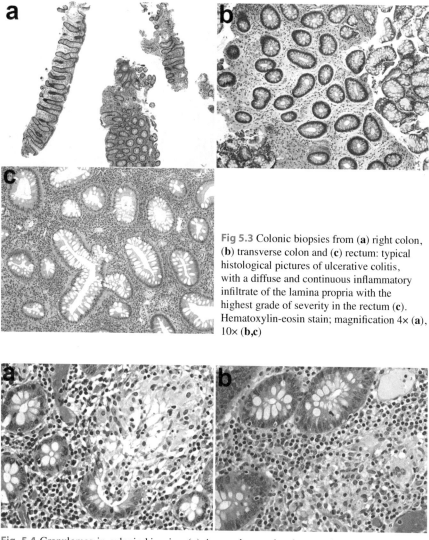

Fig 5.3 Colonic biopsies from (a) right colon, (b) transverse colon and (c) rectum: typical histological pictures of ulcerative colitis, with a diffuse and continuous inflammatory infiltrate of the lamina propria with the highest grade of severity in the rectum (c). Hematoxylin-eosin stain; magnification 4× (a), 10× (b,c)

Fig. 5.4 Granulomas in colonic biopsies. (a) A granuloma related to mucin extravasation in an active ulcerative colitis with cryptitis and gland rupture. (b) A typical granuloma of Crohn's disease, with a giant cell and not associated with gland disruption. Hematoxylin-eosin stain; magnification 40× (a,b)

increase in the chronic inflammatory infiltrate of the mucosa, even though an island of "normal-appearing" mucosa can be observed, mainly as a result of the therapy (MH), giving a patchy appearance to the colon [18, 37, 53], particularly in the rectum (rectal sparing). The extension of the disease can also change in long-standing UC, turning from diffuse and continuous to non-diffuse and discontinuous [37, 53].

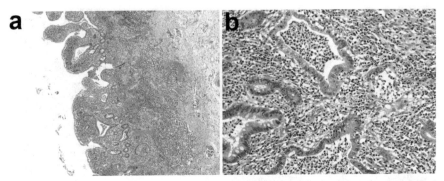

Fig. 5.5 Active ulcerative colitis: mucosal architecture distortion with gland distortion and diffuse transmucosal inflammation with basal crypt plasmacytosis. There is an evident presence of an active inflammatory component causing cryptitis and crypt abscesses with mucin depletion and gland regeneration. Of note the presence of a substantial eosinophilic component. Hematoxylin-eosin stain; magnification 4× (**a**); 20× (**b**)

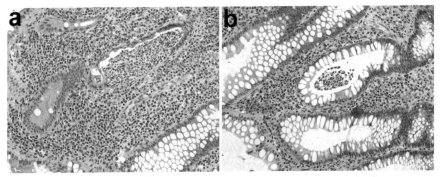

Fig. 5.6 Examples of crypt abscesses: on the left, a crypt abscess causing glandular destruction; on the right, a non-destroying crypt abscess. Hematoxylin-eosin stain; magnification 40× (**a,b**)

Therapy can also produce alterations which modify the typical histological picture until there is complete MH, which is the primary endpoint of the new guidelines [57, 58]. The pattern distribution of colitis is also modified, with a discontinuous and patchy appearance of the disease giving rise to other possible differential diagnoses, above all of Crohn's colitis (particularly in the absence of sufficient clinical data).

Histology can be used, to define a situation of chronic active or chronic inactive colitis (where signs of chronicity are found) or simply active colitis (in the absence of any signs of chronic mucosal damage).

The signs of activity (Fig. 5.5) are represented by:

- neutrophilic infiltrate in the lamina propria with the presence of cryptitis, crypt abscesses with glandular destruction (Fig. 5.6);

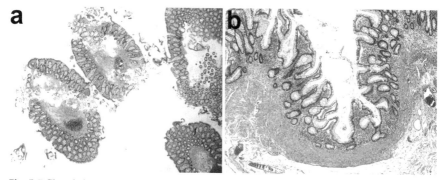

Fig. 5.7 Chronic inactive ulcerative colitis: the images show architectural distortion with glandular branching, dilatation and shortening of the crypts and glandular atrophy. Fibrosis of the lamina propria and thickening of muscularis mucosae are also visible. A mild increase in the chronic inflammatory infiltrate (with the typical basal plasmacytosis together with focal Paneth cell metaplasia) is also evident. Hematoxylin-eosin stain; magnification 2× (a), 4× (b)

- erosion/ulceration of the epithelium;
- regenerative features of the glandular cells with a reduction in mucinous cells and mucin production.

The signs of chronicity (Fig. 5.7) are:
- architectural distortion which includes branching and loss of glandular parallelism, dilatation/shortening of the crypts and/or glandular atrophy with a reduction in gland density;
- fibrosis of the lamina propria;
- reduplication and/or thickening of muscularis mucosae;
- increased chronic inflammatory cells, including basal plasmacytosis (increase in the plasmacell infiltrate along the basal region of the crypts) and/or the presence of basal lymphoid aggregates (follicular lymphoid aggregates also with a germinal center, located between the basal portion of the crypt and the muscularis mucosae;
- Paneth cell metaplasia, particularly in the left colon.

Several histological scoring systems have been created in order to analyze and compare UC histology, not only regarding the clinical management of the patients, but also regarding the purpose of clinical trials [49]. Among the most widely known and used histological classification systems (Table 5.1) are the Truelove and Richards index (which is based on a three-grade scale system) [59], Riley index (which takes into account six histological parameters, each rated on a four-point scale) [45], and the Geboes scale (which analyzes six histological features, each rated on a 0–3 or 0–4 scale) [60].

Currently, few studies exist which have correlated the histological modification and the effect of therapy in UC patients and only a few of them include alterations after biological drugs, possibly due to the late identification of this type of therapeutic agent [5].

Table 5.1 Three of the most widely used histological activity index scores

Index	Grading System	Parameters evaluated
Truelove and Richards Activity Index [59]	Three-grade scale system	Inflammatory infiltrate of the lamina propria graded from none to severe
Riley Activity Index [45]	Six parameters, each rated in a four-grade scale system (none, mild, moderate, severe)	- Neutrophilic infiltrate in the lamina propria - Crypt abscesses - Mucin depletion - Surface erosion - Chronic inflammatory cell infiltrate in the lamina propria - Crypt architectural distortion
Geboes Activity Index [60]	Six parameters (grades), each rated in a 0–3 or 0–4 scale system (subgrades)	Grade 0: architectural alteration Grade 1: chronic inflammatory infiltrate Grade 2: neutrophils (2A) and eosinophils (2B) in the lamina propria Grade 3: neutrophils in epithelium Grade 4: crypt destruction Grade 5: erosion or ulceration

5.3 Differential Diagnosis

5.3.1 Crohn's Disease and Indeterminate Colitis

The most common types of IBD which can affect the colon are UC and Crohn's Disease (CD); the distinction can be made easily if their clinical and endoscopic presentations are typical and each IBD type exhibits its classical histological features. The former is characterized by the presence of diffuse and continuous ulceration of the mucosa from the rectum to the proximal colon (the rectum is nearly always involved in non-treated UC) [61] and the latter is characterized by the presence of segmental inflammation of the intestine, with the presence of deep transmural fissuring ulcers and fistulas, aphthous mucosal erosion and granulomatous reaction [62].

Some patients, however, show features which overlap between UC and CD, and differentiating them can be difficult, especially on biopsy samples, leading the pathologist to a provisional diagnosis of "indeterminate colitis". This definition was initially coined to describe cases of fulminant colitis with colonic dilatation (i.e., toxic megacolon), proximal colon involvement and extensive ulceration of the mucosa sometimes with a fissuring appearance and marked inflammatory component extending throughout the gut wall [63]. This histological picture can be confounding since right-sided pathological disease, fissuring ulcers and transmural colonic wall inflammation are typically considered to be diagnostic of CD, but they can also be found in acute and severe UC [62, 64–67].

The pathologist should avoid the category of "indeterminate colitis" especially regarding preoperative biopsies. The European Consensus Guidelines of 2013 proposed the definition of "IBD unclassified" when the patients "clearly have inflammatory bowel disease based on the clinical history but macroscopy and/or endoscopic biopsies show no definitive features of ulcerative colitis or Crohn's disease" and underlines that this is a "temporary" definition of the disease [6]. Every attempt should be made to achieve the correct diagnosis since the treatments and surgical procedures used for UC and CD patients are different. For the most part, UC patients undergo total colectomy associated with pouch ileo-anal anastomosis (IPAA), a surgical procedure which is generally contraindicated in patients with CD due to the high risk of complications [68]. Nevertheless, some studies have demonstrated that the majority of cases of indeterminate colitis are actually cases of atypical/acute UC while 10–40% have been retrospectively proven to be Crohn's colitis [69–71]. Regardless of the diagnosis, in this acute situation, an IPAA procedure has an overall 20% risk of complications; this is intermediate between that of typical UC patients (10%) and that of CD patients (30–40%) [72, 73].

Recently, however, studies have shown the presence of UC displaying CD-like features, such as segmental disease, fissuring ulcers and appendiceal/right-sided involvement in patients with left-sided UC [61]. On the other hand, some studies have described the presence of CD limited only to the colon at the initial presentation with particular attention to a sub-group of patients in which the histological and clinical features mimic those of UC (ulcerative-like CD). In these patients, the clinical manifestations consist of total/sub-total colitis (more commonly left-sided disease in patients with ulcerative-like colitis), showing a lower percentage of strictures and stenosis, and a younger age at presentation. Histology shows superficial inflammation limited to the mucosa and submucosa, but other features more typical of CD can be found (i.e., perianal disease, skip lesions, granulomas) [61, 74].

Another confusing situation is represented by the presence of so-called "backwash ileitis" in acute and severe UC; the ileo-cecal valve allows the retrograde flow of colonic content into the distal ileum inducing a condition of inflammation which may be erroneously regarded as distal ileitis in CD [75, 76]. The presence of patchy and mild inflammation in the lamina propria (superficial inflammatory infiltrate), together with some cryptitis and regenerative aspects, are the histological features found, for the most part, without the presence of other features characteristic of CD, i.e., moderate-severe inflammatory infiltrate extending to the submucosa, granulomas, deep ulceration of the mucosa and pyloric gland metaplasia.

In conclusion, there are several situations of atypical presentation of UC:

- discontinuity in UC due to long-standing colitis in response to topical therapy or rectal sparing, in cases of good response to topical therapy or as an initial presentation, mainly in children [74];

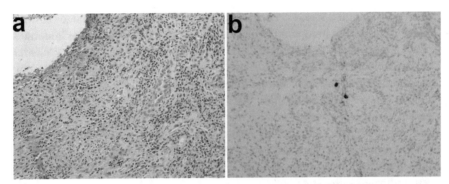

Fig. 5.8 Biopsy taken from an ulcerative colitis unresponsive to medical treatment: evident swelling and nuclear hyperchromasia of the endothelial cells of the granulation tissue. Specific immunohistochemistry against cytomegalovirus antigens is a more sensitive technique, being able to detect even a single infected cell. Hematoxylin-eosin stain; magnification 20× (**a**); Immunohistochemistry for cytomegalovirus antigens, magnification 20× (**b**)

- skip lesions with a cecal patch and/or appendiceal inflammation in left-sided UC, a recognized phenomenon which occurs mainly at presentation [77]. It should be noted that, in one study, the degree of the appendiceal inflammation was considered a predictive factor for the development of mucosal pouch inflammation [78];
- aphthous ulcers and CD-like features [61];
- backwash ileitis, mostly in the setting of acute pancolitis. The definition of this condition was proposed in 2005 by Haskell et al. [41]: they found ileal inflammation in 17% of 200 cases of colectomy, mainly limited to the last centimeter before the valve (it can be slightly longer but no more than 5 cm in length). The presence of backwash ileitis is related to the degree of right bowel inflammation or to active pancolitis. Other factors which can induce ileal inflammation are drugs (most commonly non-steroidal anti-inflammatory drugs, NSAIDs) and some bowel preparatory agents [77];
- UC displaying CD-like features;
- infections may complicate the clinical and histological pictures of UC, masking the underlying IBD. Cytomegalovirus (CMV) can cause segmental and severe flare of activity, mainly in the right colon; *Clostridium difficile* is also responsible for a flare of activity. The histology can vary from edema to pseudomembranous colitis; however, typical pseudomembranes are not the rule [79]. In cases of CMV infections, the use of immunohistochemistry can be of some help; however, histology is not a good tool for recognizing bacterial infections (Fig. 5.8).

The definition of UC has always been associated only with the involvement of the large bowel. However, recent literature has shown that UC can be found in association with inflammation of the upper gastrointestinal (GI) tract as well [80–83], making the differential diagnosis with CD (an inflammatory condition which can be found throughout the entire intestinal tract) more difficult. The real incidence of the manifestation of UC in the upper GI tract ranges from 3% to 7.6% [84, 85] and was initially found in the pediatric population (since a complete endoscopic examination is more frequently carried out in children than in adults). The histological findings are those of a diffuse mucosal inflammation, with basal plasmacytosis, crypt distortion and abscesses. A recent study by Rubenstein et al. [83] proposed the term "ulcerative colitis-associated enteritis" (UCAE). Their findings were interesting in that the inflammation of the upper GI tract becomes evident after colectomy and with the presence of an ileal pouch, and that the degree of inflammation is higher in patients with pancolitis than in those with only distal UC [86].

For the most part, other conditions and types of colitis to take into account are represented by acute self-limiting colitis, microscopic colitis and drug-induced colitis.

5.3.2   Infectious Colitis

Infectious agents are sometimes responsible for colonic mucosal damage which mimics IBD at endoscopy. The clinical picture can resemble bloody diarrhea and abdominal tenderness, with the presence of fever [87, 88]. Symptoms are usually transient and resolve within 2–4 weeks. The presence of bacterial agents in the stool is positive in only 40–60% of cases; thus, a negative result cannot exclude possible infectious colitis [87, 89].

Many infectious agents can be identified: *Entamoeba histolytica*, *Salmonella* spp., *Yersinia* spp., *Shigella* spp., *Escherichia coli*, and *Campylobacter jejuni*. The macroscopic appearance of the colonic mucosa can vary from minimal changes to a hemorrhagic, granular and friable pattern of damage. The alterations are typically not so diffuse as to involve the entire colonic mucosa even though, in the most severe cases, they can involve large segments. The right colon is more involved than the left-distal segments.

Biopsies taken at the very beginning of the disease show histological features of mucosal architectural preservation without gland distortion, edema or acute inflammatory infiltrate of the lamina propria, aspects of cryptitis with epithelial surface erosion and mucin depletion without crypt abscesses and aspects of basal cell plasmacytosis and basal lymphoid aggregates (Fig. 5.9). Granulomas are generally not a typical feature but can be found associated with ruptured glands. The presence of basal plasmacytosis has been demonstrated to be one of the most important features predictive of long-standing mucosal damage (chronic colitis) and it can thus be a reliable feature in the differential diagnosis between acute mucosal (i.e., infectious colitis) and chronic damage [51, 90].

In daily practice, however, biopsies are generally not taken in the acute phase (sometimes the endoscopy is performed after therapy), and the histological

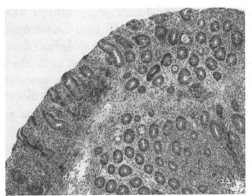

Fig. 5.9 The biopsy shows the mucosal architectural preservation without gland distortion, edema and a mixed inflammatory infiltrate of the lamina propria with mild cryptitis and focal epithelial surface erosion.
A mild mucin depletion is evident as well. Hematoxylin-eosin stain; magnification 10×

picture may show only a minimal or focal degree of mucosal inflammation with residual aspects of epithelial surface erosion or a mild increase in intraepithelial lymphocytes.

5.3.3   Diverticular Disease-associated Colitis

Diverticulosis and inflammation of colonic diverticula or diverticular disease-associated colitis (DAC) can mimic in clinical practice an early phase of IBD presenting with pain, diarrhea and rectal bleeding [91]. Histologically, IBD and DAC are very similar and almost indistinguishable; only knowledge of the distribution of the inflamed area along the bowel (i.e., sigmoidal region and rectal sparing) and information regarding the inflamed area adjacent to the diverticula can help in the differential diagnosis. It should be noted that diverticular disease and DAC are frequently found in older patients; thus, the two diseases can coexist.

5.3.4   Diversion Colitis

Diversion colitis is a term used to define inflammation of the bowel, generally the distal portion (sigmoid colon and/or rectum), caused by diversion of the fecal stream, resulting in alteration of the endoluminal bacterial environment [92]. Patients can be asymptomatic even though at the histological level, modifications can also be present. In cases of diversion colitis, the most prominent alterations to be found are typically lymphoid aggregate hyperplasia with germinal centers and mild crypt distortion, and an increase of the inflammatory cells which tend to be more pronounced in the upper part of the mucosa.

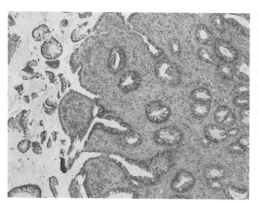

Fig. 5.10 The histological picture of colonic mucosa with ischemic features: fibrosis, mild inflammatory infiltrate of the lamina propria, and the loss of the superficial epithelium, are evident. The glands show mild atrophy and regenerative modifications. Hematoxylin-eosin stain; magnification 10×

5.3.5 Acute Ischemic Colitis

Patients present with abdominal pain, diarrhea and hematochezia; pain can be absent in 25% of patients with non-occlusive ischemic colitis. The most affected areas of the bowel are the left colon, splenic flexure and right colon. The macroscopic appearance shows superficial mucosal ulcerations (longitudinally oriented along the axis of the bowel) and pseudopolyps can be present. Histologically, the early phase shows edema, hemorrhage with a variable amount of inflammatory infiltrate of the lamina propria, the presence of necrosis, degeneration and loss of the superficial portion of the glands (Fig. 5.10). In the resolution phase, the epithelium shows regenerative modifications with an increase in chronic inflammatory cells which replace the neutrophilic component of the early phase. In cases of chronic non-occlusive disease, all the typical alterations of chronic mucosal damage can be found.

5.3.6 Radiation Colitis

In the acute phase of radiation colitis, the main changes are represented by edema, telangiectasia and fibrinoid necrosis of the small vessels. The mucosal damage is characterized by the presence of crypt abscesses with an acute inflammatory infiltrate of the lamina propria, together with a loss of glands and mucin-producing cells. Marked nuclear pleomorphism and alteration of the nuclear/cytoplasm ratio can be observed as well.

In the chronic phase, the main modifications are strictures and fistulas with superficial ulcers, and the histological features are loss of the regular gland architecture, Paneth cell metaplasia, mucosal atrophy and alteration of the vascular channels (arterial necrosis and myointimal hyperplasia).

The differential diagnosis with IBD/CD can be made mainly on the basis of the clinical setting, information regarding the past medical history of the patient and on histological features, such as basal lymph plasmacytosis, nearly always present in IBD, and non-ischemic-type mucosal ulcerations.

5.3.7 Microscopic Colitis

The definition of microscopic colitis was coined in 1980 to define clinically chronic diarrhea in an otherwise endoscopically normal colonic mucosa [93]. It ties together two distinct entities: lymphocytic colitis (LC) and collagenous colitis (CC). The former is diagnosed when a diffuse increase in the number of intra-epithelial lymphocytes (IELs) (>20 IELs/100 enterocytes) is found; the latter is based on the presence of an irregular and thicker (>10 micron) basal layer of collagen with inflammatory cells and small-sized vessels [94, 95].

One-third of cases can show histological alterations similar to those found in IBD, generally to a lesser degree. Aspects of cryptitis, crypt abscesses, minimal gland distortion, Paneth cell metaplasia and surface ulceration can also be seen in up to 44% of cases [96]. However, basal plasmacytosis and basal lymphoid aggregates are generally not present, and the inflammatory infiltrate is typically limited to the upper half of the lamina propria.

5.3.8 Drug and Preparation Solution-induced Colitis

The solutions and preparations (sodium phosphate and, less frequently, magnesium citrate) used to prepare the large bowel for endoscopy can induce mucosal alterations, such as aphthous ulcers, mainly in the distal colon [97]. Histology demonstrates superficial and focal mucosal erosions with mild-to-moderate acute inflammatory infiltrate and mild mucin depletion. Apoptotic bodies located basally in the crypts may sometimes be found together with some features of cryptitis in the absence, however, of gland destruction [98–100].

Drugs can also induce mucosal alterations and colitis which mimic IBD/UC and, of the drugs, NSAIDs are one of the most implicated. NSAID-induced colitis does not have diffuse and continuous mucosal damage but, instead, a more patchy distribution. Histology shows a milder acute inflammatory infiltrate within the lamina propria as well as a lesser degree of cryptitis.

5.4 Ulcerative Colitis and Neoplasia

5.4.1 Adenocarcinoma and Dysplasia-associated Lesion or Mass

Adenocarcinoma in UC patients has a prevalence of 3.5% and correlates with disease duration and extent [101–104], demonstrating that extensive UC has a moderate risk of developing adenocarcinoma as compared to ulcerative proctitis or only left-sided colitis. Other factors to take into account are the degree of activity of the UC, age at onset, the presence of associated primary sclerosing cholangitis (PSC) and, as expected, a positive family history of CRC [16, 105–108]. However, the real incidence of adenocarcinoma in UC is not easily evaluable since the diagnosis is influenced by numerous other factors, such as the sampling bioptic protocols, the recognition of suspicious areas, not only endoscopically but also histologically, the medical therapy and the surgical procedures used in different institutions (i.e., early colectomy in patients not responsive to medical treatment) and the methods used to detect the neoplasia. In fact, nowadays, there are new endoscopic techniques, such as chromoendoscopy, high-resolution magnification endoscopy and confocal laser endomicroscopy, which can increase the sensitivity of the detection of dysplasia/adenocarcinoma in UC patients [6].

Ulcerative colitis has an increased risk of CRC 8–10 years after onset, of approximately 0.5–1% per year [101]; therefore, it is necessary to have adequate surveillance program protocols after 8 years [109].

Dysplasia is defined according to the World Health Organization (WHO) 2010 guidelines [110] as intraepithelial neoplasia and represents the precursor lesion of CRC in all patients (general population and IBD patients). In UC, four categories can be identified: negative for dysplasia (where the glands have cytological alterations due only to regenerative aspects), indefinite for dysplasia (where the cyto-architectural glandular modifications cannot be ascribed with certainty to regenerative aspects in an otherwise active colitis background) and positive for low-grade and high-grade dysplasia. Another classification proposed and used by some centers, is the "Vienna classification" [111]; the grading system proposed is the same but, instead of the term "intraepithelial" neoplasia, the term "non-invasive" neoplasia is used.

From a histological point of view the types of dysplasia which can be recognized in UC patients are: intestinal "adenomatous" dysplasia, mucinous/villous dysplasia, serrated dysplasia and many patients frequently have a mixture of these types [91].

The features of intestinal dysplasia include mucosal thickening, architectural gland crowding, cigar-shape and elongation of enterocytes with an altered nuclear-cytoplasm ratio, nuclear hyperchromasia, nuclear overlapping and stratification with mitotic figures and mucin depletion [112]. Mucinous dysplasia generally has a villiform pattern with a mucin-rich epithelium and basally-oriented nuclei with little cytological atypia. The serrated type of dysplasia is similar to a sessile serrated adenoma found in the general population, with a saw-like appearance of the glands, a predominance of non-goblet cells and eosinophilic cytoplasm with nuclear enlargement and prominent nucleoli [91].

Interobserver agreement is high for the categories of negative and high-grade dysplasia, but there is poor agreement regarding the indefinite and low-grade dysplasia categories; according to the European Consensus Guidelines 2013, statement 17, "Confirmation of dysplasia by an independent expert GI pathologist is recommended" [6]. Immunohistochemistry for P53 and

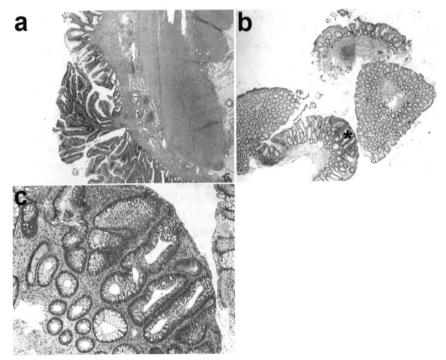

Fig 5.11 Examples of dysplasia in ulcerative colitis. **a** An example of DALM (dysplasia-associated lesion or mass), non-adenoma-like in a colectomy specimen. The patient underwent colon resection due to the presence of an endoscopically unresectable velvety mucosal plaque. **b** An example of flat dysplasia, found incidentally during random biopsies taken in the follow-up. At a higher magnification the area of intestinal dysplasia shows the features of classic intestinal dysplasia (*asterisk*) with mucosal thickening, architectural gland crowding, cigar shape and elongation of enterocytes with an altered nuclear-cytoplasm ratio, nuclear hyperchromasia, overlapping and stratification and mucin depletion. Hematoxylin-eosin stain; magnification 2× (**a,b**), magnification 20× (**c**)

alpha-methylacyl-CoA racemase (AMACR) can support the pathologist in the diagnosis: P53 is overexpressed in dysplastic glands and the epithelium [113, 114], and AMACR has an increasing positive gradient in colonic glands, from low-grade dysplasia to adenocarcinoma [115, 116].

According to the European Consensus Guidelines (statement 19), the surveillance follow-up of UC patients should include "4 biopsy specimens taken from every 10 cm of the entire colon in addition to biopsies from macroscopically visible atypical lesions".

In UC, two patterns of dysplasia can be detected (Fig. 5.11): flat dysplasia and elevated dysplasia (the so-called DALM, dysplasia-associated lesion or mass). The former is generally not visible endoscopically and is diagnosed on random biopsies; the latter includes the adenoma-like lesions and non-adenoma-like lesions [117, 118].

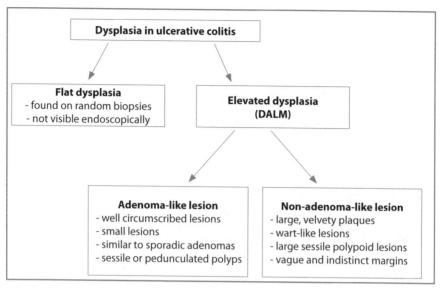

Fig 5.12 Dysplasia found in ulcerative colitis

From a morphological point of view, adenoma and non-adenoma-like lesions can be differentiated by the presence of a more heterogeneous appearance in the latter case, with a mixture of non-dysplastic and neoplastic glands, and with foci of dysplasia in the surrounding flat mucosa [118–120]. The adenoma-like lesions are sharply demarcated without foci of dysplasia in the adjacent mucosa and resemble the sporadic adenomas found in the general population (Fig. 5.12). The distinction between these two forms is important because the management of the patient is different (statement 19 of the European Consensus Guidelines).

High-grade dysplasia in flat lesions has proven to be associated with CRC, and CRC can be found in 42–67% of patients with high-grade flat dysplasia [102, 119]. Conversely, general agreement on the management of patients with low-grade dysplasia has not yet been reached and, even now, the decision to perform a colectomy is personalized and discussed with the patient [102]. Studies have demonstrated that low-grade dysplasia has a 9-fold higher risk of developing CRC than non-dysplastic colonic mucosa; on the other hand, other studies have shown that, although there is an increased risk to progression, none of the patients with low-grade dysplasia evolved to high-grade dysplasia or CRC after up to 10 years of mean follow-up [121, 122]. Left-sided low-grade dysplasia has been proven to progress more rapidly to CRC than proximally located low-grade dysplasia [123].

Adenoma-like lesions in UC can be treated with a polypectomy as are sporadic adenomas in the general population. On the contrary, non-adenoma-like lesions in UC patients represent a high risk for malignancy and, thus, colectomy should be considered [119, 124].

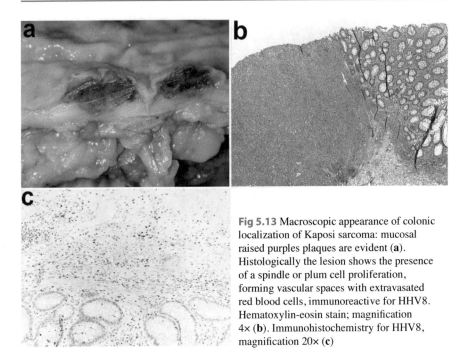

Fig 5.13 Macroscopic appearance of colonic localization of Kaposi sarcoma: mucosal raised purples plaques are evident (**a**). Histologically the lesion shows the presence of a spindle or plum cell proliferation, forming vascular spaces with extravasated red blood cells, immunoreactive for HHV8. Hematoxylin-eosin stain; magnification 4× (**b**). Immunohistochemistry for HHV8, magnification 20× (**c**)

5.4.2 Lymphoma and Ulcerative Colitis

Lymphoproliferative disorders do not have increased incidence in UC patients as compared to the general population; some studies have found a variable percentage ranging from 3% to 15% of cases [125, 126]. In all those cases, the diagnosis was not clinically suspected since the clinical picture presented as a worsening of the symptoms and a non-response to therapy [127]. In UC patients, lymphoproliferative disorders are most frequently multifocal and located in the distal portion of the colon, mainly in areas of active colitis [128, 129]. In the general population, lymphoproliferative disorders are more frequent in the cecum and ascending colon.

5.4.3 Kaposi Sarcoma

Kaposi Sarcoma (KS) is caused by human herpesvirus-8 (HHV8) infection and only a few cases associated with UC have been reported in the literature, mainly related to refractory UC where continuous steroid therapy is required. Clinically, KS presents with signs and symptoms mimicking an acute flair of UC (diarrhea and rectal bleeding) [130] and skin lesions may occasionally be present as well. The lack of skin lesions makes the diagnosis even more challenging. The relationship between the dosage or duration of the steroid therapy and KS has not yet been clarified [131] nor has the association between UC duration and KS [132].

Macroscopically, KS presents as a vascular lesion with raised purple plaques. Histologically, it is composed of spindle or plump cell proliferation, with mild cytological atypia, forming vascular spaces which contain extravasated erythrocytes. Strong nuclear immunoreactivity of these cells for HHV8 confirms the diagnosis (Fig. 5.13).

5.5   Complications

5.5.1   Pouchitis

Total colectomy is the surgical procedure for UC and involves intestinal luminal restoration with an ileal pouch-anal anastomosis. In this situation, the ileal mucosa of the pouch undergoes adaptive changes to the new intestinal microbiota environment which is evidenced at histology by a mild increase in the acute inflammatory infiltrate (both neutrophils and eosinophils) in the lamina propria with, mild villous atrophy, an increase in Paneth cells and a partial transition to a more colonic mucin phenotype [133]. Therefore, the diagnosis of pouchitis should be made taking into consideration these histological modifications and only in the presence of an appropriate clinical and endoscopic setting.

Ulcerative colitis patients can experience pouchitis with an incidence which increases with the length of the follow-up (60–80% in the first 5 years after surgery in a more than 10-year follow-up) [134–136]. The study of Yantiss et al. demonstrated that at least one episode of pouchitis was experienced in approximately 50% of patients in the first year after colectomy [137]; nevertheless, fewer than 1% of patients required removal of the pouch [138].

The etiology of this ileal mucosa inflammation remains unclear; it is not a consequence of the surgical procedure since it does not usually appear in non-IBD patients (i.e., patients who undergo total colectomy for familial adenomatous polyposis) [91], and it does not seem to be associated with the presence of backwash ileitis [139]. The clinical symptoms are variable ranging from an increase in bowel movements (occasionally associated with bloody diarrhea, malaise and fever) to tenesmus or fecal incontinence. In some cases, patients can develop perianal fistulas or abscesses.

Macroscopically, the mucosa of the pouch can present as granular with a hemorrhagic and friable pattern, and with ulcers and superficial erosions. The histological features are an increase in the inflammatory infiltrate, which is mainly neutrophilic in the acute or chronic-active form or is mainly composed of lympho-mononuclear cells in the chronic type. The ileal mucosa can show varying degrees of atrophy, erosion and ulcers. Distortion of the mucosal

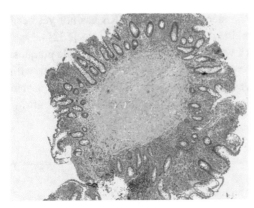

Fig. 5.14 Pouchitis: the ileal mucosa shows features of "colonization" with varying degrees of glandular atrophy, epithelial erosion and ulcers. There is increase of the inflammatory infiltrate and mild mucosal architecture distortion. Hematoxylin-eosin stain; magnification 4×

architecture, pyloric gland metaplasia, increased number of Paneth cells and fibrosis of the lamina propria can be seen mainly in the chronic and recurrent forms (Fig. 5.14). Features of "colonization" of the ileal mucosa can be seen and represent adaptative changes with a change to a more "colonic phenotype" of the glands [140]. These modifications can be divided into three patterns [141]:
1. ileal mucosa retaining its typical villous architecture;
2. flattening of the mucosa with a chronic inflammatory infiltrate of the lamina propria;
3. inflamed mucosa with phases of activity alternating with phases of recovery.

Occasionally, granulomas associated with rupture of the mucinous glands can be observed, and transmural inflammation can also occur. All these inflammatory alterations can lead to stenosis and fistula, a picture which could raise the suspicion of CD. However, granulomas are not the signature of CD since they can also be related to foreign material (sutures) or infective agents, and transmural inflammation can also be seen in pouchitis not responsive to antibiotic therapy [91].

Studies have demonstrated that histology is less sensitive in grading pouchitis than endoscopy or a clinical activity index. In 1994 Sandborn et al. developed a pouchitis scoring system which is not commonly used in clinical practice at present [142]; nevertheless, it is widely used in association with endoscopy to evaluate concomitant events, such as co-infections or ischemia.

Infective agents are among the most frequent causes of pouchitis, and the most common pathogens are represented by *Clostridium difficile*, *Shigella* spp., *Escherichia coli* and CMV [91]. Unfortunately, infective-based pouchitis does not have typical features, being similar to the inflammation which can occur in a non-IBD patient having a moderate acute inflammatory infiltrate of the lamina propria with glandular and surface epithelial erosion and aggression; for the most part, the diagnosis is reached by means of a positive stool culture. A differential diagnosis with ischemia is easily reached; the histological features of the ischemic pouch are the same as those observed in any other tract of the gut, typically with disruption of the muscular cells of the muscularis mucosae and with fibrosis of the lamina propria.

Diagnosing CD based on a pouch specimen is very challenging; however, it must be considered when non-necrotizing granulomas (not in association with ruptured crypts or glands) and/or deep penetrating fistulas are seen at histology. In this situation, revision of the slides concerning the colectomy specimen and/or previous biopsy specimens is necessary before changing the diagnosis from UC to CD.

5.5.2 Cuffitis

Cuffitis is the inflammation of the residual columnar mucosa, or "cuff", of the rectum left behind (that which is not totally removed during the IPAA surgical procedure) and proximally located to the anal canal. Cuffitis occurs in up to 13% of patients [143]. The symptoms can mimic those of pouchitis; however, the diagnosis is easily reached by endoscopic examination; the mucosa of the cuff rather than that of the ileal pouch is inflamed.

5.5.3 Pre-pouch Ileitis

This condition is defined by the presence of chronic inflammation of the ileal tract proximal to the neo-pouch in patients with IPAA with or without concomitant pouchitis [144]. The histological changes are the same as those observed for pouchitis with the presence of a more colonic appearance of the small intestinal glands (with a mucin and phenotypic modification).

5.5.4 Crohn's Disease-like Complications of the Pouch

A newly described inflammatory complication involving the ileal pouch after IPAA for UC has been called Crohn's disease-like (CD-like) pouchitis. It affects up to 13% of patients and it manifests in the afferent ileal limb (pre-pouch) as non-anastomotic strictures/stenosis or with non-anastomotic peri-anal fistula [145, 146]. At histology a diffuse acute inflammatory infiltrate of the lamina propria can be observed as well as the presence of erosion, ulceration and mucosal architecture distortion. In surgical excision of the pouch, deep lymphoid aggregates can be seen together with fistulas lined by granulation tissue [147].

A recent study by Huguet et al. [148] showed higher efficacy in the use of the anti-tumor necrosis factor (TNF) drugs in CD-like complications than in chronic refractory pouchitis, suggesting different triggers and mechanisms sustaining the two inflammatory conditions. The former is related to a possible "de novo CD of the pouch", as suggested by some authors [149, 150], and the latter is more related to "microbiota-mediated" inflammation, as observed by some studies [151, 152] and confirmed by the greater efficacy of the use of antibiotics and by the lesser response to anti-TNF therapy [153, 154].

5.6   Infections

5.6.1   Cytomegalovirus

Cytomegalovirus is a double-stranded DNA virus which causes either acute infection or the reactivation of latent infections in immunocompromised patients. According to the European Guideline 2013 [6], UC patients have a greater risk of this opportunistic infection than CD patients [155]; the drug and therapeutic regimen of the patients may greatly influence the risk of infection together with a situation of "steroid-refractory" UC. Cytomegalovirus over-infection causes an increased severity of UC disease, and a higher risk of morbidity and hospitalization; CMV infection must be ruled out whenever UC becomes unresponsive to medical treatment and, in any case, before starting a more aggressive immunosuppressive therapy [156–158]. Several studies have demonstrated the efficacy of anti-CMV therapy in patients, thus decreasing the need for surgical colectomy/proctocolectomy and inducing clinical remission [159].

From a histological point of view, CMV infection causes morphological alterations, such as swelling and nuclear hyperchromasia with nuclear body inclusions, mainly in endothelial cells [160]. However, these findings are not always present on simple hematoxylin-eosin stained slides; specific immunohistochemistry against CMV antigens is a more sensitive technique, being able to detect even a single infected cell (Fig. 5.8).

5.6.2   Clostridium difficile

Clostridium difficile is a spore-forming bacterium with a wide spectrum of clinical presentation, ranging from watery diarrhea and abdominal pain to toxic megacolon and perforation. In patients with ileostomy, *C. difficile* infection may cause enteritis and in those with an IPAA, the infection can be responsible for pouchitis (in up to 10.7% of cases) [161]. In UC patients, the incidence of *C. difficile* ranges from 2.8% to 11% [162], and long-term therapy with corticosteroids and immunomodulator agents together with antibiotics has been demonstrated to have an increased risk for *C. difficile* infection [163, 164]. On the contrary, no relationship with the recent introduction of the biological agents into clinical practice has been demonstrated [165]. According to the study by Navaneethan at al., the risk factors for *C. difficile* infection in UC patients are represented by severe endoscopic disease activity, a high number of emergency room visits within a 3-month period, an elevated number of hospitalizations and escalation in medication within 1 year from hospitalization. In addition, these patients, are more likely to have a higher number of ER visits in the first year after the infection as compared to non-infected patients and a higher risk of colectomy as well [166].

The histological features are not specific in the majority of cases, merely showing active colitis since only 13% of UC patients present with pseudomembrane at endoscopy [91].

5.7   Ulcerative Colitis in Children

Approximately 10–15% of UC patients are children under 18 years of age [167]. The gold standard for diagnosis is endoscopic evaluation of the lower and upper gastrointestinal tracts with biopsies for histological confirmation [168–170]. At presentation, UC in children is more frequently extensive colitis (total or sub-total colitis) with features of backwash ileitis and peri-appendiceal inflammation, also in cases without severe cecal UC involvement [6]. Nevertheless, the histological picture of UC in children can be more challenging than in adults; the colonic mucosa may show a lesser degree of distortion, preserving the regular architecture in up to 31% of cases. The inflammation can be mild and patchy (approximately 21% of cases) and rectal sparing can be detected (approximately 30%), especially in children under 10 years of age [34, 35, 171, 172].

As reported by some studies, basal cell plasmacytosis is not so common in children as compared to UC in adults (58%) but, when present, it represents an early event even in young children [35, 172]. The inflammation of the upper GI tract can be seen in up to 75% of pediatric patients [173–175] as non-specific esophagitis or gastritis; conversely, duodenal mucosa inflammation is not common [175, 176].

References

1. Stange EF, Travis SPL, Vermeire S et al; European Crohn's and Colitis Organisation (ECCO) (2008) European evidence-based Consensus on the diagnosis and management of ulcerative colitis: definitions and diagnosis. J Crohns Colitis 2(1):1–23
2. Mowat C, Cole A, Windsor A et al; IBD Section of the British Society of Gastroenterology (2011) Guidelines for the management of inflammatory bowel disease in adults. Gut 60(5):571–607

3. Delpre G, Avidor I, Steinherz R et al (1989) Ultrastructural abnormalities in endoscopically and histologically normal and involved colon in ulcerative colitis. Am J Gastroenterol 84(9):1038–1046

4. Geboes K, Dalle I (2002) Influence of treatment on morphological features of mucosal inflammation. Gut 50 (Suppl 3):III37–III42

5. Wiernicka A, Szymanska S, Cielecka-Kuszyk J et al (2015) Histological healing after infliximab induction therapy in children with ulcerative colitis. World J Gastroenterol 21(37):10654–10661

6. Magro F, Langner C, Driessen A et al; European Society of Pathology (ESP); European Crohn's and Colitis Organisation (ECCO) (2013) European consensus on the histopathology of inflammatory bowel disease. J Crohns Colitis 7(10):827–851

7. Truelove SC, Hambling MH (1958) Treatment of ulcerative colitis with local hydrocortisone hemisuccinate sodium: a report on a controlled therapeutic trial. Br Med J 2(5104):1072–1077

8. Thomas SJ, Walsh A, Von Herbay A et al (2009) How much agreement is there between histological, endoscopic and clinical assessments of remission in ulcerative colitis? Gut 58(S1):A101

9. Rosenberg L, Nanda KS, Zenlea T et al (2013) Histologic markers of inflammation in patients with ulcerative colitis in clinical remission. Clin Gastroenterol Hepatol 11(8): 991–996

10. Moum B, Ekbom A, Vatn MH, Elgjo K (1999) Change in the extent of colonoscopic and histological involvement in ulcerative colitis over time. Am J Gastroenterol 94(6):1564–1569

11. Levine TS, Tzardi M, Mitchell S et al (1996) Diagnostic difficulty arising from rectal recovery in ulcerative colitis. J Clin Pathol 49(4):319–323

12. Rubio CA, Johansson C, Uribe A, Kock Y (1984) A quantitative method of estimating inflammation in the rectal mucosa. IV. Ulcerative colitis in remission. Scand J Gastroenterol 19(4):525–530

13. Price AB, Morson BC (1975) Inflammatory bowel disease: the surgical pathology of Crohn's disease and ulcerative colitis. Hum Pathol 6(1):7–29

14. Mazzuoli S, Guglielmi FW, Antonelli E et al (2013) Definition and evaluation of mucosal healing in clinical practice. Dig Liver Dis 45(12):969–977

15. Gupta RB, Harpaz N, Itzkowitz S et al (2007) Histologic inflammation is a risk factor for progression to colorectal neoplasia in ulcerative colitis: a cohort study. Gastroenterology 133(4):1099–1105

16. Rutter M, Saunders B, Wilkinson K et al (2004) Severity of inflammation is a risk factor for colorectal neoplasia in ulcerative colitis. Gastroenterology 126(2):451–459

17. Bitton A, Peppercorn MA, Antonioli DA et al (2001) Clinical, biological, and histologic parameters as predictors of relapse in ulcerative colitis. Gastroenterology 120(1):13–20

18. Schumacher G, Kollberg B, Sandstedt B (1994) A prospective study of first attacks of inflammatory bowel disease and infectious colitis. Histologic course during the 1st year after presentation. Scand J Gastroenterol 29(4):318–332

19. Azad S, Sood N, Sood A (2011) Biological and histological parameters as predictors of relapse in ulcerative colitis: a prospective study. Saudi J Gastroenterol 17(3):194–198

20. Korelitz BI, Sultan K, Kothari M et al (2014) Histological healing favors lower risk of colon carcinoma in extensive ulcerative colitis. World J Gastroenterol 20(17):4980–4986

21. Hefti MM, Chessin DB, Harpaz NH et al (2009) Severity of inflammation as a predictor of colectomy in patients with chronic ulcerative colitis. Dis Colon Rectum 52(2):193–197

22. Tanaka M, Saito H, Kusumi T et al (2002) Biopsy pathology predicts patients with ulcerative colitis subsequently requiring surgery. Scand J Gastroenterol 37(2):200–205

23. Tanaka M, Kusumi T, Oshitani N et al (2003) Validity of simple mucosal biopsy criteria combined with endoscopy predicting patients with ulcerative colitis ultimately requiring surgery: a multicenter study. Scand J Gastroenterol 38(6):594–598

24. Zezos P, Patsiaoura K, Nakos A et al (2014) Severe eosinophilic infiltration in colonic biopsies predicts patients with ulcerative colitis not responding to medical therapy. Colorectal Dis 16(12):O420–O430
25. Daperno M, Sostegni R, Scaglione N et al (2004) Outcome of a conservative approach in severe ulcerative colitis. Dig Liver Dis 36(1):21–28
26. Molnár T, Farkas K, Nyári T et al (2011) Response to first intravenous steroid therapy determines the subsequent risk of colectomy in ulcerative colitis patients. J Gastrointestin Liver Dis 20(4):359–363
27. Travis SPL, Higgins PDR, Orchard T et al (2011) Review article: defining remission in ulcerative colitis. Aliment Pharmacol Ther 34(2):113–124
28. Bryant RV, Winer S, Travis SP, Riddell RH (2014) Systematic review: histological remission in inflammatory bowel disease. Is 'complete' remission the new treatment paradigm? An IOIBD initiative. J Crohns Colitis 8(12):1582–1597
29. Conrad K, Roggenbuck D, Laass MW (2014) Diagnosis and classification of ulcerative colitis. Autoimmun Rev 13(4–5):463–466
30. Geboes K, Desreumaux P, Jouret A et al (1999) Histopathologic diagnosis of the activity of chronic inflammatory bowel disease. Evaluation of the effect of drug treatment. Use of histological scores. Gastroenterol Clin Biol 23(10):1062–1073 [Article in French]
31. Sanders DS (1998) The differential diagnosis of Crohn's disease and ulcerative colitis. Baillieres Clin Gastroenterol 12(1):19–33
32. Swan NC, Geoghegan JG, O'Donoghue DP et al (1998) Fulminant colitis in inflammatory bowel disease: detailed pathologic and clinical analysis. Dis Colon Rectum 41(12):1511–1515
33. Palnaes Hansen C, Hegnhøj J, Møller A et al (1990) Ulcerative colitis and Crohn's disease of the colon. Is there a macroscopic difference? Ann Chir Gynaecol 79(2):78–81
34. Glickman JN, Bousvaros A, Farraye FA et al (2004) Pediatric patients with untreated ulcerative colitis may present initially with unusual morphologic findings. Am J Surg Pathol 28(2):190–197
35. Washington K, Greenson JK, Montgomery E et al (2002) Histopathology of ulcerative colitis in initial rectal biopsy in children. Am J Surg Pathol 26(11):1441–1449
36. Joo M, Odze RD (2010) Rectal sparing and skip lesions in ulcerative colitis: a comparative study of endoscopic and histologic findings in patients who underwent proctocolectomy. Am J Surg Pathol 34(5):689–696
37. Kim B, Barnett JL, Kleer CG, Appelman HD (1999) Endoscopic and histological patchiness in treated ulcerative colitis. Am J Gastroenterol 94(11):3258–3262
38. D'Haens G, Geboes K, Ponette E et al (1997) Healing of severe recurrent ileitis with azathioprine therapy in patients with Crohn's disease. Gastroenterology 112(5):1475–1481
39. Ladefoged K, Munck LK, Jorgensen F, Engel P (2005) Skip inflammation of the appendiceal orifice: a prospective endoscopic study. Scand J Gastroenterol 40(10):1192–1196
40. Yang SK, Jung HY, Kang GH et al (1999) Appendiceal orifice inflammation as a skip lesion in ulcerative colitis: an analysis in relation to medical therapy and disease extent. Gastrointest Endosc 49(6):743–747
41. Haskell H, Andrews CW Jr, Reddy SI et al (2005) Pathologic features and clinical significance of "backwash" ileitis in ulcerative colitis. Am J Surg Pathol 29(11):1472–1481
42. Koukoulis GK, Ke Y, Henley JD, Cummings OW (2002) Detection of pyloric metaplasia may improve the biopsy diagnosis of Crohn's ileitis. J Clin Gastroenterol 34(2):141–143
43. Goldstein N, Dulai M (2006) Contemporary morphologic definition of backwash ileitis in ulcerative colitis and features that distinguish it from Crohn disease. Am J Clin Pathol 126(3):365–376
44. Yamagata M, Mikami T, Tsuruta T et al (2011) Submucosal fibrosis and basic-fibroblast growth factor-positive neutrophils correlate with colonic stenosis in cases of ulcerative colitis. Digestion 84(1):12–21
45. Riley SA, Mani V, Goodman MJ et al (1991) Microscopic activity in ulcerative colitis: what does it mean? Gut 32(2):174–178

46. Villanacci V, Manenti S, Antonelli E et al (2011) Non-IBD colitides: clinically useful histopathological clues. Rev Esp Enferm Dig 103(7):366–372
47. Baars JE, Nuij VJ, Oldenburg B et al (2012) Majority of patients with inflammatory bowel disease in clinical remission have mucosal inflammation. Inflamm Bowel Dis 18(9):1634–1640
48. Bessissow T, Lemmens B, Ferrante M et al (2012) Prognostic value of serologic and histologic markers on clinical relapse in ulcerative colitis patients with mucosal healing. Am J Gastroenterol 107(11):1684–1692
49. Mosli MH, Feagan BG, Sandborn WJ et al (2014) Histologic evaluation of ulcerative colitis: a systematic review of disease activity indices. Inflamm Bowel Dis 20(3):564–575
50. Surawicz CM, Meisel JL, Ylvisaker T et al (1981) Rectal biopsy in the diagnosis of Crohn's disease: value of multiple biopsies and serial sectioning. Gastroenterology 80(1):66–71
51. Surawicz CM, Haggitt RC, Husseman M, McFarland LV (1994) Mucosal biopsy diagnosis of colitis: acute self-limited colitis and idiopathic inflammatory bowel disease. Gastroenterology 107(3):755–763
52. McCormick DA, Horton LW, Mee AS (1990) Mucin depletion in inflammatory bowel disease. J Clin Pathol 43(2):143–146
53. Kleer CG, Appelman HD (1998) Ulcerative colitis: patterns of involvement in colorectal biopsies and changes with time. Am J Surg Pathol 22(8):983–989
54. Cross SS, Harrison RF (2002) Discriminant histological features in the diagnosis of chronic idiopathic inflammatory bowel disease: analysis of a large dataset by a novel data visualisation technique. J Clin Pathol 55(1):51–57
55. Gramlich T, Petras RE (2007) Pathology of inflammatory bowel disease. Semin Pediatr Surg 16(3):154–163
56. Mahadeva U, Martin JP, Patel NK, Price AB (2002) Granulomatous ulcerative colitis: a re-appraisal of the mucosal granuloma in the distinction of Crohn's disease from ulcerative colitis. Histopathology 41(1):50–55
57. Odze R, Antonioli D, Peppercorn M, Goldman H (1993) Effect of topical 5-aminosalicylic acid (5-ASA) therapy on rectal mucosal biopsy morphology in chronic ulcerative colitis. Am J Surg Pathol 17(9):869–875
58. Kornbluth A, Sachar DB; Practice Parameters Committee of the American College of Gastroenterology (2004) Ulcerative colitis practice guidelines in adults (update): American College of Gastroenterology, Practice Parameters Committee. Am J Gastroenterol 99(7):1371–1385
59. Truelove SC, Richards WC (1956) Biopsy studies in ulcerative colitis. Br Med J 1(4979):1315–1318
60. Geboes K, Riddell R, Ost A et al (2000) A reproducible grading scale for histological assessment of inflammation in ulcerative colitis. Gut 47(3):404–409
61. Soucy G, Wang HH, Farraye FA et al (2012) Clinical and pathological analysis of colonic Crohn's disease, including a subgroup with ulcerative colitis-like features. Mod Pathol 25(2):295–307
62. Odze RD (2003) Diagnostic problems and advances in inflammatory bowel disease. Mod Pathol 16(4):347–358
63. Odze RD (2004) Pathology of indeterminate colitis. J Clin Gastroenterol 38(5 Suppl 1):S36–S40
64. Geboes K (2001) Crohn's disease, ulcerative colitis or indeterminate colitis – how important is it to differentiate? Acta Gastroenterol Belg 64(2):197–200
65. Goldman H (1998) Ulcerative colitis and Crohn's disease. In: Ming S, Goldman H (eds) Pathology of the gastrointestinal tract. Williams & Wilkins, Baltimore, pp. 673–694
66. Yantiss RK, Farraye FA, O'Brien MJ et al (2006) Prognostic significance of superficial fissuring ulceration in patients with severe 'indeterminate' colitis. Am J Surg Pathol 30(2):165–170
67. Guindi M, Riddell RH (2004) Indeterminate colitis. J Clin Pathol 57(12):1233–1244

68. Braveman JM, Schoetz DJ Jr, Marcello PW et al (2004) The fate of the ileal pouch in patients developing Crohn's disease. Dis Colon Rectum 47(10):1613–1619
69. Yu CS, Pemberton JH, Larson D (2000) Ileal pouch-anal anastomosis in patients with indeterminate colitis: long-term results. Dis Colon Rectum 43(11):1487–1496
70. Farmer M, Petras RE, Hunt LE et al (2000) The importance of diagnostic accuracy in colonic inflammatory bowel disease. Am J Gastroenterol 95(11):3184–3188
71. Meucci G, Bortoli A, Riccioli FA et al (1999) Frequency and clinical evolution of indeterminate colitis: a retrospective multi-centre study in northern Italy. GSMII (Gruppo di Studio per le Malattie Infiammatorie Intestinali). Eur J Gastroenterol Hepatol 11(8):909–913
72. Panis Y, Poupard B, Nemeth J et al (1996) Ileal pouch/anal anastomosis for Crohn's disease. Lancet 347(9005):854–857
73. Peyrègne V, Francois Y, Gilly FN et al (2000) Outcome of ileal pouch after secondary diagnosis of Crohn's disease. Int J Colorectal Dis 15(1):49–53
74. Feakins RM (2014) Ulcerative colitis or Crohn's disease? Pitfalls and problems. Histopathology 64(3):317–335
75. McCready FJ, Bargen JA, Dockerty MB et al (1949) Involvement of the ileum in chronic ulcerative colitis. N Engl J Med 240(4):119–127
76. Saltzstein SL, Rosenberg BF (1963) Ulcerative colitis of the ileum, and regional enteritis of the colon: a comparative histopathologic study. Am J Clin Pathol 40:610–623
77. Yantiss RK, Odze RD (2007) Pitfalls in the interpretation of nonneoplastic mucosal biopsies in inflammatory bowel disease. Am J Gastroenterol 102(4):890–904
78. Yantiss RK, Sapp HL, Farraye FA et al (2004) Histologic predictors of pouchitis in patients with chronic ulcerative colitis. Am J Surg Pathol 28(8):999–1006
79. Yantiss RK, Odze RD (2006) Diagnostic difficulties in inflammatory bowel disease pathology. Histopathology 48(2):116–132
80. Lin J, McKenna BJ, Appelman HD (2010) Morphologic findings in upper gastrointestinal biopsies of patients with ulcerative colitis: a controlled study. Am J Surg Pathol 34(11):1672–1677
81. Vidali F, Di Sabatino A, Broglia F et al (2010) Increased CD8+ intraepithelial lymphocyte infiltration and reduced surface area to volume ratio in the duodenum of patients with ulcerative colitis. Scand J Gastroenterol 45(6):684–689
82. Endo K, Kuroha M, Shiga H et al (2012) Two cases of diffuse duodenitis associated with ulcerative colitis. Case Rep Gastrointest Med 2012:396521 doi:10.1155/2012/396521
83. Rubenstein J, Sherif A, Appelman H, Chey WD (2004) Ulcerative colitis associated enteritis: is ulcerative colitis always confined to the colon? J Clin Gastroenterol 38(1):46–51
84. Hisabe T, Matsui T, Miyaoka M et al (2010) Diagnosis and clinical course of ulcerative gastroduodenal lesion associated with ulcerative colitis: possible relationship with pouchitis. Dig Endosc 22(4):268–274
85. Hori K, Ikeuchi H, Nakano H et al (2008) Gastroduodenitis associated with ulcerative colitis. J Gastroenterol 43(3):193–201
86. Honma J, Mitomi H, Murakami K et al (2001) Nodular duodenitis involving CD8+ cell infiltration in patients with ulcerative colitis. Hepatogastroenterology 48(42):1604–1610
87. Nostrant TT, Kumar NB, Appelman HD (1987) Histopathology differentiates acute self-limited colitis from ulcerative colitis. Gastroenterology 92(2):318–328
88. Surawicz CM (2008) What's the best way to differentiate infectious colitis (acute self-limited colitis) from IBD? Inflamm Bowel Dis 14(Suppl 2):S157–S158
89. Kumar NB, Nostrant TT, Appelman HD (1982) The histopathologic spectrum of acute self-limited colitis (acute infectious-type colitis). Am J Surg Pathol 6(6):523–529
90. Seldenrijk CA, Morson BC, Meuwissen SG et al (1991) Histopathological evaluation of colonic mucosal biopsy specimens in chronic inflammatory bowel disease: diagnostic implications. Gut 32(12):1514–1520

91. Odze RD, Goldblum JR (2015) Surgical pathology of the GI tract, liver, biliary tract and pancreas (3rd edn). Elsevier Saunders, Philadelphia
92. Morson BC, Dawson IMP (1972) Gastrointestinal pathology. Blackwell, Oxford-London
93. Read NW, Krejs GJ, Read MG et al (1980) Chronic diarrhea of unknown origin. Gastroenterology 78(2):264–271
94. Lazenby AJ, Yardley JH, Giardiello FM et al (1989) Lymphocytic ("microscopic") colitis – a comparative histopathologic study with particular reference to collagenous colitis. Hum Pathol 20(1):18–28
95. Bo-Linn GW, Vendrell DD, Lee E, Fordtran JS (1985) An evaluation of the significance of microscopic colitis in patients with chronic diarrhea. J Clin Invest 75(5):1559–1569
96. Ayata G, Ithamukkala S, Sapp H et al (2002) Prevalence and significance of inflammatory bowel disease-like morphologic features in collagenous and lymphocytic colitis. Am J Surg Pathol 26(11):1414–1423
97. NASPGHAN/CCFA Working Group (2007) Differentiating ulcerative colitis from Crohn disease in children and young adults: report of a working group of the North American Society for Pediatric Gastroenterology, Hepatology, and Nutrition and the Crohn's and Colitis Foundation of America. J Pediatr Gastroenterol Nutr 44(5):653–674
98. Driman DK, Preiksaitis HG (1998) Colorectal inflammation and increased cell proliferation associated with oral sodium phosphate bowel preparation solution. Hum Pathol 29(9):972–978
99. Watts DA, Lessells AM, Penman ID, Ghosh S (2002) Endoscopic and histologic features of sodium phosphate bowel preparation induced colonic ulceration: case report and review. Gastrointest Endosc 55(4):584–587
100. Wong NA, Penman ID, Campbell S, Lessells AM (2000) Microscopic focal cryptitis associated with sodium phosphate bowel preparation. Histopathology 36(5):476–478
101. Bergeron V, Vienne A, Sokol H et al (2010) Risk factors for neoplasia in inflammatory bowel disease patients with pancolitis. Am J Gastroenterol 105(11):2405–2411
102. Farraye FA, Odze RD, Eaden J, Itzkowitz SH (2010) AGA technical review on the diagnosis and management of colorectal neoplasia in inflammatory bowel disease. Gastroenterology 138(2):746–774
103. Lashner BA (2002) Colorectal cancer surveillance for patients with inflammatory bowel disease. Gastrointest Endosc Clin N Am 12(1):135–143
104. Ullman T, Odze R, Farraye FA (2009) Diagnosis and management of dysplasia in patients with ulcerative colitis and Crohn's disease of the colon. Inflamm Bowel Dis 15(4):630–638
105. Broomé U, Löfberg R, Veress B, Eriksson LS (1995) Primary sclerosing cholangitis and ulcerative colitis: evidence for increased neoplastic potential. Hepatology 22(5):1404–1408
106. Mooiweer E, Baars JE, Lutgens MW et al (2012) Disease severity does not affect the interval between IBD diagnosis and the development of CRC: results from two large, Dutch case series. J Crohns Colitis 6(4):435–440
107. Nuako KW, Ahlquist DA, Mahoney DW et al (1998) Familial predisposition for colorectal cancer in chronic ulcerative colitis: a case-control study. Gastroenterology 115(5):1079–1083
108. Askling J, Dickman PW, Karlén P et al (2001) Family history as a risk factor for colorectal cancer in inflammatory bowel disease. Gastroenterology 120(6):1356–1362
109. Rutter MD, Saunders BP, Wilkinson KH et al (2006) Thirty-year analysis of a colonoscopic surveillance program for neoplasia in ulcerative colitis. Gastroenterology 130(4):1030–1038
110. Bosman FT, Carneiro F, Hruban RH, Theise ND (2010) WHO classification of tumours of the digestive system (4th edn). WHO Press, Lyon
111. Schlemper RJ, Riddell RH, Kato Y et al (2000) The Vienna classification of gastrointestinal epithelial neoplasia. Gut 47(2):251–255

112. Riddell RH, Goldman H, Ransohoff DF et al (1983) Dysplasia in inflammatory bowel disease: standardized classification with provisional clinical applications. Hum Pathol 14(11):931–968
113. Gerrits MM, Chen M, Theeuwes M et al (2011) Biomarker-based prediction of inflammatory bowel disease-related colorectal cancer: a case-control study. Cell Oncol (Dordr) 34(2):107–117
114. Pozza A, Scarpa M, Ruffolo C et al (2011) Colonic carcinogenesis in IBD: molecular events. Ann Ital Chir 82(1):19–28
115. Dorer R, Odze RD (2006) AMACR immunostaining is useful in detecting dysplastic epithelium in Barrett's esophagus, ulcerative colitis, and Crohn's disease. Am J Surg Pathol 30(7):871–877
116. van Schaik FD, Oldenburg B, Offerhaus GJ et al (2012) Role of immunohistochemical markers in predicting progression of dysplasia to advanced neoplasia in patients with ulcerative colitis. Inflamm Bowel Dis 18(3):480–488
117. Odze RD (1999) Adenomas and adenoma-like DALMs in chronic ulcerative colitis: a clinical, pathological, and molecular review. Am J Gastroenterol 94(7):1746–1750
118. Torres C, Antonioli D, Odze RD (1998) Polypoid dysplasia and adenomas in inflammatory bowel disease: a clinical, pathologic, and follow-up study of 89 polyps from 59 patients. Am J Surg Pathol 22(3):275–284
119. Rutter MD, Saunders BP, Wilkinson KH et al (2004) Most dysplasia in ulcerative colitis is visible at colonoscopy. Gastrointest Endosc 60(3):334–339
120. Vieth M, Behrens H, Stolte M (2006) Sporadic adenoma in ulcerative colitis: endoscopic resection is an adequate treatment. Gut 55(8):1151–1155
121. Lim CH, Dixon MF, Vail A et al (2003) Ten year follow up of ulcerative colitis patients with and without low grade dysplasia. Gut 52(8):1127–1132
122. Befrits R, Ljung T, Jaramillo E, Rubio C (2002) Low-grade dysplasia in extensive, long-standing inflammatory bowel disease: a follow up study. Dis Colon Rectum 45(5): 615–620
123. Goldstone R, Itzkowitz S, Harpaz N, Ullman T (2011) Progression of low-grade dysplasia in ulcerative colitis: effect of colonic location. Gastrointest Endosc 74(5):1087–1093
124. Blackstone MO, Riddell RH, Rogers BH, Levin B (1981) Dysplasia associated lesion or mass (DALM) detected by colonoscopy in long-standing ulcerative colitis: an indication for colectomy. Gastroenterology 80(2):366–374
125. Fan CW, Changchien CR, Wang JY et al (2000) Primary colorectal lymphoma. Dis Colon Rectum 43(9):1277–1282
126. Shepherd NA, Hall PA, Coates PJ, Levison DA (1988) Primary malignant lymphoma of the colon and rectum. A histopathological and immunohistochemical analysis of 45 cases with clinicopathological correlations. Histopathology 12(3):235–252
127. Holubar SD, Dozois EJ, Loftus EV Jr et al (2011) Primary intestinal lymphoma in patients with inflammatory bowel disease: a descriptive series from the prebiologic therapy era. Inflamm Bowel Dis 17(7):1557–1563
128. Lenzen R, Borchard F, Lübke H, Strohmeyer G (1995) Colitis ulcerosa complicated by malignant lymphoma: case report and analysis of published works. Gut 36(2):306–310
129. Wong NA, Herbst H, Herrmann K et al (2003) Epstein-Barr virus infection in colorectal neoplasms associated with inflammatory bowel disease: detection of the virus in lymphomas but not in adenocarcinomas. J Pathol 201(2):312–318
130. Querido S, Sousa HS, Pereira TA et al (2015) Gastrointestinal bleeding and diffuse skin thickening as Kaposi sarcoma clinical presentation. Case Rep Transplant 2015:424508
131. Anderson LA, Lauria C, Romano N et al (2008) Risk factors for classical Kaposi sarcoma in a population-based case-control study in Sicily. Cancer Epidemiol Biomarkers Prev 17(12):3435–3443
132. Rodríguez-Peláez M, Fernández-García MS, Gutiérrez-Corral N et al (2010) Kaposi's sarcoma: an opportunistic infection by human herpesvirus-8 in ulcerative colitis. J Crohns Colitis 4(5):586–590

133. Cremonini F, Talley NJ (2005) Irritable bowel syndrome: epidemiology, natural history, health care seeking and emerging risk factors. Gastroenterol Clin North Am 34(2): 189–204
134. Ikeuchi H, Nakano H, Uchino M et al (2004) Incidence and therapeutic outcome of pouchitis for ulcerative colitis in Japanese patients. Dig Surg 21(3):197–201
135. Suzuki H, Ogawa H, Shibata C et al (2012) The long-term clinical course of pouchitis after total proctocolectomy and IPAA for ulcerative colitis. Dis Colon Rectum 55(3):330–336
136. Meier CB, Hegazi RA, Aisenberg J et al (2005) Innate immune receptor genetic polymorphisms in pouchitis: is CARD15 a susceptibility factor? Inflamm Bowel Dis 11(11):965–971
137. Yantiss RK, Sapp HL, Farraye FA et al (2004) Histologic predictors of pouchitis in patients with chronic ulcerative colitis. Am J Surg Pathol 28(8):999–1006
138. Rotimi O, Rodrigues MG, Lim C (2004) Microscopic colitis with giant cells: is it really a distinct pathological entity? Histopathology 44(5):503–505
139. Araki T, Hashimoto K, Okita Y et al (2018) Colonic histological criteria predict development of pouchitis after ileal pouch-anal anastomosis for patients with ulcerative colitis. Dig Surg 35(2):138–143
140. Biancone L, Palmieri G, Lombardi A et al (2003) Tropomyosin expression in the ileal pouch: a relationship with the development of pouchitis in ulcerative colitis. Am J Gastroenterol 98(12):2719–2726
141. Fruin AB, El-Zammer O, Stucchi AF et al (2003) Colonic metaplasia in the ileal pouch is associated with inflammation and is not the result of long-term adaptation. J Gastrointest Surg 7(2):246–253
142. Le Berre N, Heresbach D, Kerbaol M et al (1995) Histological discrimination of idiopathic inflammatory bowel disease from other types of colitis. J Clin Pathol 48(8):749–753
143. Thompson-Fawcett MW, Mortensen NJ, Warren BF (1999) "Cuffitis" and inflammatory changes in the columnar cuff, anal transitional zone, and ileal reservoir after stapled pouch-anal anastomosis. Dis Colon Rectum 42(3):348–355
144. Bell AJ, Price A, Forbes A et al (2006) Pre-pouch ileitis: a disease of the ileum in ulcerative colitis after restorative proctocolectomy. Colorectal Dis 8(5):402–410
145. Shen B, Fazio VW, Remzi FH, Lashner BA (2005) Clinical approach to diseases of ileal pouch-anal anastomosis. Am J Gastroenterol 100(12):2796–2807
146. Samaan MA, de Jong D, Sahami S et al (2016) Incidence and severity of prepouch ileitis: A distinct disease entity or a manifestation of refractory pouchitis? Inflamm Bowel Dis 22(3):662–668
147. Warren BF, Shepherd NA, Bartolo DC, Bradfield JW (1993) Pathology of the defunctioned rectum in ulcerative-colitis. Gut 34(4):514–516
148. Huguet M, Pereira B, Goutte M et al (2018) Systematic review with meta-analysis: anti-TNF therapy in refractory pouchitis and Crohn's disease-like complications of the pouch after ileal pouch-anal anastomosis following colectomy for ulcerative colitis. Inflamm Bowel Dis 24(2):261–268
149. Goldstein NS, Sanford WW, Bodzin JH (1997) Crohn's-like complications in patients with ulcerative colitis after total proctocolectomy and ileal pouch-anal anastomosis. Am J Surg Pathol 21(11):1343–1353
150. Deutsch AA, McLeod RS, Cullen J, Cohen Z (1991) Results of the pelvic-pouch procedure in patients with Crohn's disease. Dis Colon Rectum 34(6):475–477
151. Cheifetz A, Itzkowitz S (2004) The diagnosis and treatment of pouchitis in inflammatory bowel disease. J Clin Gastroenterol 38(5 Suppl 1):S44–S50
152. Angriman I, Scarpa M, Castagliuolo I (2014) Relationship between pouch microbiota and pouchitis following restorative proctocolectomy for ulcerative colitis. World J Gastroenterol 20(29):9665–9674
153. Colombel JF, Sandborn WJ, Rutgeerts P et al (2007) Adalimumab for maintenance of clinical response and remission in patients with Crohn's disease: the CHARM trial. Gastroenterology 132(1):52–65

154. Holubar SD, Cima RR, Sandborn WJ, Pardi DS (2010) Treatment and prevention of pou-chitis after ileal pouch-anal anastomosis for chronic ulcerative colitis. Cochrane Database Syst Rev 2010(6):CD001176
155. Pillet S, Pozzetto B, Jarlot C et al (2012) Management of cytomegalovirus infection in inflammatory bowel diseases. Dig Liver Dis 44(7):541–548
156. Kim JJ, Simpson N, Klipfel N et al (2010) Cytomegalovirus infection in patients with active inflammatory bowel disease. Dig Dis Sci 55(4):1059–1065
157. Kim YS, Kim YH, Kim JS et al; IBD Study Group of the Korean Association for the Study of Intestinal Diseases(KASID), Korea (2012) Cytomegalovirus infection in patients with new onset ulcerative colitis: a prospective study. Hepatogastroenterology 59(116):1098–1101
158. Roblin X, Pillet S, Oussalah A et al (2011) Cytomegalovirus load in inflamed intestinal tissue is predictive of resistance to immunosuppressive therapy in ulcerative colitis. Am J Gastroenterol 106(11):2001–2008
159. Kambham N, Vij R, Cartwright CA, Longacre T (2004) Cytomegalovirus infection in steroid-refractory ulcerative colitis: a case-control study. Am J Surg Pathol 28(3):365–373
160. Sinzger C (2008) Entry route of HCMV into endothelial cells. J Clin Virol 41(3):174–179
161. Li Y, Qian J, Queener E, Shen B (2013) Risk factors and outcome of PCR-detected Clostridium difficile infection in ileal pouch patients. Inflamm Bowel Dis 19(2):397–403
162. D'Aoust J, Battat R, Bessissow T (2017) Management of inflammatory bowel disease with Clostridium difficile infection. World J Gastroenterol 23(27):4986–5003
163. Rodemann JF, Dubberke ER, Reske KA et al (2007) Incidence of Clostridium difficile infection in inflammatory bowel disease. Clin Gastroenterol Hepatol 5(3):339–344
164. Issa M, Vijayapal A, Graham MB et al (2007) Impact of Clostridium difficile on inflammatory bowel disease. Clin Gastroenterol Hepatol 5(3):345–351
165. Schneeweiss S, Korzenik J, Solomon DH et al (2009) Infliximab and other immunomodu-lating drugs in patients with inflammatory bowel disease and the risk of serious bacterial infections. Aliment Pharmacol Ther 30(3):253–264
166. Navaneethan U, Mukewar S, Venkatesh PG et al (2012) Clostridium difficile infection is associated with worse long term outcome in patients with ulcerative colitis. J Crohns Colitis 6(3):330–336
167. Kugathasan S, Judd RH, Hoffmann RG et al; Wisconsin Pediatric Inflammatory Bowel Disease Alliance (2003) Epidemiologic and clinical characteristics of children with newly diagnosed inflammatory bowel disease in Wisconsin: a statewide population-based study. J Pediatr 143(4):525–531
168. Dubinsky M (2008) Special issues in pediatric inflammatory bowel disease. World J Gastroenterol 14(3):413–420
169. Gupta SK, Fitzgerald JF, Croffie JM et al (2004) Comparison of serological markers of inflammatory bowel disease with clinical diagnosis in children. Inflamm Bowel Dis 10(3):240–244
170. Kim SC, Ferry GD (2004) Inflammatory bowel diseases in pediatric and adolescent pa-tients: clinical, therapeutic, and psychosocial considerations. Gastroenterology 126(6): 1550–1560
171. Markowitz J, Kahn E, Grancher K et al (1993) Atypical rectosigmoid histology in children with newly diagnosed ulcerative colitis. Am J Gastroenterol 88(12):2034–2037
172. Robert ME, Tang L, Hao LM, Reyes-Mugica M (2004) Patterns of inflammation in mucosal biopsies of ulcerative colitis – perceived differences in pediatric populations are limited to children younger than 10 years. Am J Surg Pathol 28(2):183–189
173. Abdullah BA, Gupta SK, Croffie JM et al (2002) The role of esophagogastroduodenoscopy in the initial evaluation of childhood inflammatory bowel disease: a 7-year study. J Pediatr Gastroenterol Nutr 35(5):636–640
174. Ruuska T, Vaajalahti P, Arajärvi P, Mäki M (1994) Prospective evaluation of upper gastrointestinal mucosal lesions in children with ulcerative colitis and Crohn's disease. J Pediatr Gastroenterol Nutr 19(2):181–186

175. Sharif F, McDermott M, Dillon M et al (2002) Focally enhanced gastritis in children with Crohn's disease and ulcerative colitis. Am J Gastroenterol 97(6):1415–1420
176. Kundhal PS, Stormon MO, Zachos M et al (2003) Gastral antral biopsy in the differentiation of pediatric colitides. Am J Gastroenterol 98(3):557–561

Medical Treatment of Ulcerative Colitis: Does Traditional Therapy Still Have a Role?

6

Fernando Rizzello, Marco Salice, Carlo Calabrese, Marta Mazza, Andrea Calafiore, Lucia Calandrini, Hana Privitera Hrustemovic, Massimo Campieri, and Paolo Gionchetti

6.1 Introduction and Definitions

Ulcerative colitis (UC) is a chronic inflammatory disease which involves the colonic mucosa continuously starting from the rectum and progressively involving the entire colon. Its etiology is still unknown, although numerous studies have clarified the inflammatory mechanisms involved in the pathogenesis, allowing the development of new targeted drugs.

Correct medical treatment requires the evaluation of disease extension, activity and behavior [1].

The Montreal classification allows extent to be defined into three subgroups: proctitis (when the inflammation is limited to the rectum), left-sided colitis (distal to the splenic flexure), and extensive or pancolitis (proximal to the splenic flexure) [2]. Drug formulation is chosen based on the disease extent: suppositories for proctitis, enemas for left-sided colitis and tablets for extensive colitis. Furthermore, patients with extensive colitis have a higher risk of colectomy or of developing colorectal cancer, justifying the need for strict disease control and histological surveillance [3–5].

Many disease activity indices have been proposed, but none has been adequately validated; the Truelove and Witts clinical index and the Mayo composite score are the scores most used in clinical trials. In clinical practice, the Truelove and Witts score is used mainly to identify a severe relapse while the Mayo score is used in mild-to-moderate activity (Tables 6.1 and 6.2) [6, 7].

F. Rizzello (✉)
Department of Medical and Surgical Sciences, University of Bologna, S. Orsola-Malpighi Hospital
Bologna, Italy
e-mail: fernando.rizzello@unibo.it

G. Poggioli (Ed), *Ulcerative Colitis,*
Updates in Surgery
DOI: 10.1007/978-88-470-3977-3_6, © Springer-Verlag Italia 2019

Table 6.1 The Truelove and Witts index

	Mild	Moderate*	Severe
Bloody stools/day	<4	4 or more *If*	≥6 *and*
Pulse	<90 bpm	≤90 bpm	>90 bpm *or*
Temperature	<37.5°C	≤37.8°C	>37.8°C *or*
Hemoglobin	>11.5 g/dl	≥10.5 g/dl	<10.5 g/dl *or*
ESR	<20 mm/h	≤30 mm/h	>30 mm/h

* Moderate: between mild and severe
ESR, erythrocyte sedimentation rate

Table 6.2 The Mayo score

	Stool frequency	Rectal bleeding	Endoscopic findings	Physician global assessment
0	Normal number of stools for this patient	No blood seen	Normal or inactive disease	Normal
1	1–2 stools more than normal	Streaks of blood in the stool less than half the time	Erythema, decreased vascular pattern, mild friability	Mild disease
2	3–4 stools more than normal	Obvious blood in the stool most of the time	Marked erythema, absent vascular pattern, friability, erosions	Moderate disease
3	5 or more stools more than normal	Only blood passed	Spontaneous bleeding, ulcerations	Severe disease

The major limitation of the Truelove and Witts severity index is that it is not sufficiently discriminative to measure changes in disease activity.

The Mayo score is a composite quantitative score ranging from 0 to 12 points, divided into 3 clinical items plus the endoscopic findings. The definition of remission, response and worsening is not uniform in the different studies and none of these definitions has been formally validated. Studies evaluating the efficacy of biological drugs in active UC have defined: *clinical remission* as a total Mayo score of ≤2 points with no individual subscore >1 point; *clinical response* as a decrease from baseline in the total Mayo score of ≥3 points and ≥30%, and a decrease in the rectal bleeding subscore of ≥1 point or an absolute rectal bleeding subscore of 0 or 1; and *mucosal healing* as an absolute endoscopy subscore of 0 or 1 [8–12].

The definition of refractoriness is crucial in order to avoid side effects, overtreatment and a delay in disease control. Treatment refractoriness must

be defined after checking the correct dosage, duration, formulation, patient compliance and complications. Patients will be defined as treatment-refractory in the case of active disease despite:
- mesalamine at a correct dosage and formulation after 2–4 weeks;
- oral prednisone or methylprednisolone 0.75–1 mg/kg after 2 weeks [13];
- intravenous (IV) hydrocortisone 400 mg or methylprednisolone 1 mg/kg IV after 3–5 days [13];
- azathioprine (AZA) 2.5 mg/kg or 6-mercaptopurine (6-MP) 1.5 mg/kg after 3 months [13];
- cyclosporine 2 mg/kg IV after 4–7 days [13];
- infliximab (IFX), adalimumab (ADA), golimumab (GOLI), vedolizumab (VEDO) after 4–10 weeks [8–12 2×].

Steroid dependency is defined as a disease relapse during the 3-month dosage tapering or 3 months of steroid weaning [13].

6.2   Management of Mild-to-moderate Activity

5-aminosalicylic acid (5-ASA), also called mesalamine, the active anti-inflammatory part of sulfasalazine introduced in inflammatory bowel disease (IBD) treatment by Nana Svartz in the 1930s, is the first-line treatment for mild-to-moderate active UC [14]. The different formulations, such as suppositories, enemas and tablets, and different dosages and release mechanisms allow administering the drug directly to the inflamed area, optimizing efficacy and limiting side effects [15].

Steroids could also traditionally be administered orally and topically [16]. The introduction of oral and topical low-bioavailability steroids – such as beclomethasone dipropionate (BDP) or budesonide (BUDE) – improved safety and maintained efficacy [17–25]. The combination treatment using mesalamine and BDP has been demonstrated to be more effective than either one alone [26]. However, steroids are used mainly in cases of mesalamine refractoriness or intolerance.

6.2.1   Proctitis

The first-line therapy for active mild-to-moderate proctitis involves mesalamine suppositories 1 g once daily for 6–8 weeks [27]. Numerous studies and systematic reviews have demonstrated that mesalamine suppositories:
- are more effective than a placebo or oral mesalamine formulation [28];
- better tolerated than enemas [29];
- given in a single administration have similar efficacy to a divided dose and are better tolerated [30].

Topical steroids are less effective than topical mesalamine and are recommended for patients refractory to mesalamine [31].

The association between oral and topical mesalamine formulation or topical mesalamine and topical steroids is more effective than either one alone but, also in this case, the combination treatment is recommended only in refractory patients [32].

In cases of refractoriness to mesalamine plus steroid topical combination therapy, systemic corticosteroids, biologics and/or immunosuppressors are indicated [33].

6.2.2   Left-sided and Extensive Colitis

Oral plus topical mesalamine is the first-line therapy in active mild-to-moderate left-sided UC. The combined route is more effective than oral or topical alone [32], and both are superior to placebo [31, 32, 34].

No conclusive data are available comparing the efficacy of topical mesalamine and topical steroids but mesalamine seems to be superior to traditional steroids [31] and equivalent to topical BDP [35].

No differences have been reported in terms of efficacy between different topical mesalamine dosages (1, 2, or 4 g) [36]; however, despite the fact that no differences have been reported when comparing different enema volumes and liquids, or foam enemas, in clinical practice enemas capable of covering the entire disease extension are recommended.

A dosage of ≥2 g/day of oral mesalamine is more effective than a lower dosage [34], except in cases of moderate activity where a higher dosage of 4.8 g/day is recommended [37].

Mesalamine is as effective as sulfasalazine but is better tolerated, in particular at higher dosages [3]. Sulfasalazine maintains its role in patients with associated spondyloarthropathies. A once-daily dose is more effective than divided doses with better compliance and similar side effects [38–40].

In clinical practice, additional therapy should be started if no clinical benefit is obtained after 2 weeks of treatment, while 4–8 weeks of treatment are required in order to have complete clinical and endoscopic remission [40, 41].

As previously mentioned, in cases of mesalamine failure, the combination of topical mesalamine plus topical steroids is recommended [32]. Oral BDP 5 mg/day for 4 weeks instead of systemic corticosteroids could be a valid add-on therapy in patients refractory to mesalamine [19, 42].

Oral BUDE 9 mg MMX formulation for 8 weeks was tested in two controlled clinical trials for mild active left-sided and extensive UC. BUDE was significantly superior to a placebo in both studies but not superior to mesalamine 2.4 g/day and non-MMX BUDE 9 mg/day [43, 44]. When BUDE was used as add-on therapy in patients not adequately controlled by mesalamine 2.4 g/day, it was significantly more effective than a placebo [45].

In clinical practice, BDP and BUDE could be used for patients refractory to mesalamine as an alternative and before using systemic steroids in cases of multi-refractoriness.

Systemic steroids are superior to mesalamine in patients with extensive colitis [46, 47]. Baron proposed steroid dosages in the 1960s in a small study comparing three different dosages of prednisolone: 40 mg per day was as efficacious as 60 mg and had a better safety profile, similar to 20 mg per day [48].

6.3   Management of Severe Activity

Management of a patient with severe active UC is independent of the disease extent. In the past, severe active UC was a life-threatening disease and death occurred in almost 30% of episodes until the introduction of the intensive intravenous steroid regimen by Truelove in the 1970s [49].

After hospital admission, a patient's medical history must be carefully collected and any infective complications must be ruled out. A joint medical and surgical evaluation is strongly recommended. Intravenous steroids (hydrocortisone 400 mg/day or methylprednisolone 0.75–1 mg/kg/day) as a bolus injection [50] are the mainstays of treatment for severe active UC but the possibility of an urgent colectomy must be evaluated (i.e., in cases of perforation, septic complications, toxic megacolon or a history of repeated severe attacks) [49].

No data are available regarding the correct steroid dosage or type of steroids; however, a meta-analysis seemed to suggest that the risk of colectomy is independent of steroid dosage [51].

Other measures are:
- fluid and electrolyte supplementation as needed;
- nutritional support mainly in malnourished patients and possibly by enteral rather than parenteral nutrition. The initial concept of bowel rest has been superseded [52], and enteral nutrition is associated with fewer side effects than parenteral nutrition [53];
- topical therapy with mesalamine or corticosteroids, or both [49];
- broad spectrum antibiotics mainly when a systemic infection is suspected since they are not effective in improving the disease outcome [54–56];
- blood or albumin transfusion;
- subcutaneous prophylactic low-molecular-weight heparin in order to reduce the risk of thromboembolism [57].

Travis et al. demonstrated that, after 3 days of steroid treatment, patients with >8 bloody stools per day or between 3 and 8 bloody stools per day and C-reactive protein >45 mg/l had an 85% risk of colectomy [58]. Based on these data, called the Oxford criteria, rescue therapy should be started earlier.

Lichtiger first proposed rescue therapy in patients with active severe UC who failed to respond to intravenous corticosteroids. Intravenous cyclosporine 4 mg/ kg was tested in a small open-label study precociously interrupted because of the strongly positive results [59] Two subsequent consecutive studies showed that IV cyclosporine 4 mg/kg/day was as effective as IV cyclosporine 2 mg/kg/day [60] and that IV cyclosporine 4 mg/kg/day was as effective as IV methylprednisolone 40 mg/day [61]. Numerous small open-label studies have confirmed the efficacy of cyclosporine but have also reported infectious complications causing a patient's death. Pooling the data of these studies, cyclosporine is effective in 76–85% of patients in order to avoid colectomy in the short term. The major problem of cyclosporine treatment is the ineffectiveness of maintaining remission [62–64]. Combining it with AZA improves the maintenance of remission [65], tapering steroids and switching to oral cyclosporine 5–8 mg/kg/day until the thiopurine takes effect. When combining three immunosuppressors, such as steroids, cyclosporine and AZA, the risk of severe and life-threatening infection is higher than when using a single drug.

In the biological era, IFX has been demonstrated to be as effective as rescue therapy in steroid-refractory severe active UC patients. Jarnerot has demonstrated that a single dose of IFX 5 mg/kg is more effective than a placebo in avoiding colectomy for 3 months. [66]. Other studies have suggested that a three-dose induction is more effective in preventing colectomy [67], mainly reducing the duration of the induction period [68]. When comparing IFX and cyclosporine, both drugs are equally effective, rapid and safe [69, 70] but IFX is more effective in maintaining remission [71].

Based on the data obtained by pooling the results of 10 studies regarding third-line rescue therapy, Narula et al. recently suggested that this method is possible (28.3% colectomy rate at 3 months and 42.3% at 12 months) with an acceptable risk (6.7% serious infections and 1% mortality) [72, 73]. However, this approach should be reserved for highly selected patients in a tertiary referral center [74].

6.4   Maintenance of Remission

The main outcome of maintenance treatment is clinical and mucosal remission without steroids. Oral mesalamine at a dosage of at least 2 g once daily is the first-line treatment in patients who responded to mesalamine during the induction phase [34]. Selected patients with proctitis or left-sided colitis may be treated with topical mesalamine (suppositories or enemas, respectively) 3 g/week alone or combined with oral mesalamine in cases of inefficacy of the former alone [33].

Thiopurines are indicated at a dosage of 2–2.5 mg/kg/day for AZA or 1–1.5 mg/kg/day for 6-MP in patients refractory or intolerant to mesalamine, patients who experienced a moderate-to-severe relapse who required steroids and/ or cyclosporine or tacrolimus, and patients who were steroid-dependent. The evidence supporting the use of thiopurines as a maintenance treatment in UC is of poor quality and comes from retrospective series. The major problems in thiopurine treatment is poor tolerability and action slowness, requiring 3 months before the effectiveness can be judged, using steroids or cyclosporine as a bridge therapy [75–78].

6.5 Special Situations

The identification of the tumor necrosis factor (TNF) as a pivotal key of the inflammatory process and the introduction of monoclonal antibodies – also called "biologics", based on in vivo biotechnological production – as a therapeutic option in chronic inflammatory diseases has profoundly modified the treatment of UC.

In fact, patients with chronically active moderate UC refractory or intolerant to steroids could also be treated with IFX (5 mg/kg IV at week 0, 2 and 6) or ADA (160 mg subcutaneously at week 0 and 80 mg at week 2) or GOLI (200 mg subcutaneously at week 0 and 100 mg at week 2) [8–13]. All these monoclonal antibodies are more effective in inducing and maintaining clinical response than a placebo, but no head-to-head studies could help in identifying the best monoclonal antibodies. Furthermore, they are effective in maintaining remission at different administration schedules (Table 6.3).

Patients who failed to respond to a first anti-TNF course were defined as "primary failure", and treatment with VEDO should be considered.

Patients who lost the clinical response, mainly because they developed neutralizing anti-drug antibodies, could regain the response by optimizing the dosage used (10 mg/kg instead of 5 mg/kg) [79] or reducing the schedule interval (every 4 weeks instead of 8 weeks), or both, during IFX treatment or by reducing the schedule interval (weekly treatment) during ADA treatment [80]. No dosage optimization was used during GOLI treatment. In this case, a switch to VEDO is also possible [81]. In cases of allergic reaction or other drug-related side-effects (i.e., paradoxical psoriasis), switching to VEDO is mandatory [81].

Integrins are pivotal molecules involved in the process in which leukocytes move from the circulation to the site of inflammation; VEDO is a monoclonal antibody against alpha4-beta7 integrin expressed mainly in the endothelium of the intestinal vessels. As previously mentioned, VEDO is also effective in inducing and maintaining clinical response in patients with moderate-to-severe UC.

Table 6.4 summarizes the efficacy in the induction and maintenance of IFX, ADA, GOLI and VEDO. Once again, in this case, no head-to-head studies are available to help clinicians choose between TNF-blockers and VEDO.

Table 6.3 Administration schedule of biologics

	Route	Induction	Maintenance
Infliximab	IV	5 mg/kg at weeks 0, 2, 6	5 mg/kg every 8 weeks or 10 mg/kg every 4–8 weeks *
Adalimumab	SC	160 mg at week 0–80 mg at week 2	40 mg every other week or 40 mg every week*
Golimumab	SC	200 mg at week 0–100 mg at week 2	50 mg /4 weeks for body weight <80 kg 100 mg/4 weeks for body weight >80 kg
Vedolizumab	IV	300 mg at weeks 0, 2, 6	300 mg every 8 weeks or 300 mg every 4 weeks*

IV, intravenous; *SC*, subcutaneous
* in case of secondary failure.

Table 6.4 Efficacy of biologics in inducing and maintaining remission in patients with moderate-to-severe ulcerative colitis (no head-to-head studies)

	Route	Anti-TNF expressed	Response at induction (%)	Response at 1 year (%)
Infliximab	IV	No	ACT 1: 69% ACT 2: 64%	ACT 1: 38.8%
Adalimumab	SC	ULTRA 1: YES ULTRA 2: YES	ULTRA 1: 54.65% ULTRA 2: 50.4%	ULTRA 2: 30.2%
Golimumab	SC	PURSUIT: YES PURSUIT-M: YES	PURSUIT: 51%	PURSUIT-M: 100 mg/4 weeks: 49.7% 50 mg/4 weeks: 47%
Vedolizumab	IV	YES	VEDO: 47.1%	VEDO E8W: 56.6% VEDO E4W: 52%

TNF, tumor necrosis factor; *IV*, intravenous; *SC*, subcutaneous.

References

1. Dignass A, Eliakim R, Magro F et al (2012) Second European evidence-based consensus on the diagnosis and management of ulcerative colitis. Part 1: Definitions and diagnosis. J Crohns Colitis 6(10):965–990
2. Silverberg MS, Satsangi J, Ahmad T et al (2005) Toward an integrated clinical, molecular and serological classification of inflammatory bowel disease: report of a Working Party of the 2005 Montreal World Congress of Gastroenterology. Can J Gastroenterol 19(Suppl A): 5A –36A
3. Koutroubakis IE, Regueiro M, Schoen RE et al (2016) Multiyear patterns of serum inflammatory biomarkers and risk of colorectal neoplasia in patients with ulcerative colitis. Inflamm Bowel Dis 22(1):100–105
4. Kleer CG, Appelman HD (1998) Ulcerative colitis: patterns of involvement in colorectal biopsies and changes with time. Am J Surg Pathol 22(8):983–989
5. Magro F, Langner C, Driessen A et al; European Society of Pathology (ESP); European Crohn's and Colitis Organisation (ECCO) (2013) European consensus on the histopathology of inflammatory bowel disease. J Crohns Colitis 7(10):827–851

6. Truelove SC, Witts LJ (1955) Cortisone in ulcerative colitis. Final report on a therapeutic trial. Br Med J 2(4947):1041–1048
7. Schroeder KW, Tremaine WJ, Ilstrup DM (1987) Coated oral 5-aminosalicylic acid therapy for mildly to moderately active ulcerative colitis. A randomized study. N Engl J Med 317(26):1625–1629
8. Rutgeerts P, Sandborn WJ, Feagan BG et al (2005) Infliximab for induction and maintenance therapy for ulcerative colitis. N Engl J Med 353(23):2462–2476
9. Reinisch W, Sandborn WJ, Hommes DW et al (2011) Adalimumab for induction of clinical remission in moderately to severely active ulcerative colitis: results of a randomised controlled trial. Gut 60(6):780–787
10. Sandborn WJ, van Assche G, Reinisch W et al (2012) Adalimumab induces and maintains clinical remission in patients with moderate-to-severe ulcerative colitis. Gastroenterology 142(2):257–265
11. Sandborn WJ, Feagan BG, Marano C et al; PURSUIT-SC Study Group (2014) Subcutaneous golimumab induces clinical response and remission in patients with moderate-to-severe ulcerative colitis. Gastroenterology 146(1):85–95
12. Sandborn WJ, Feagan BG, Marano C et al; PURSUIT-Maintenance Study Group (2014) Subcutaneous golimumab maintains clinical response in patients with moderate-to-severe ulcerative colitis. Gastroenterology 146(1):96–109
13. Feagan BG, Rutgeerts P, Sands BE et al; GEMINI 1 Study Group (2013) Vedolizumab as induction and maintenance therapy for ulcerative colitis. N Engl J Med 369(8):699–710
14. Svartz N (1942) Salazopyrin, a new sulfanilamide preparation. A. Therapeutic results in rheumatic polyarthritis. B. Therapeutic results in ulcerative colitis. C. Toxic manifestations in treatment with sulfanilamide preparations. Acta Med Scand 110(6):577–598
15. Gionchetti P, Rizzello F, Annese V et al; Italian Group for the Study of Inflammatory Bowel Disease (IG-IBD) (2017) Use of corticosteroids and immunosuppressive drugs in inflammatory bowel disease: clinical practice guidelines of the Italian group for the study of inflammatory bowel disease. Dig Liver Dis 49(6):604–617
16. Stein RB, Hanauer SB (2000) Comparative tolerability of treatments for inflammatory bowel disease. Drug Saf 23(5):429–448
17. Truelove SC (1960) Systemic and local corticosteroids therapy in ulcerative colitis. Br Med J 1(5171):464–467
18. Rizzello F, Gionchetti P, Galeazzi R et al (2001) Oral beclomethasone dipropionate in patients with mild to moderate ulcerative colitis: a dose-finding study. Adv Ther 18(6):216–271
19. Rizzello F, Gionchetti P, D'Arienzo A et al (2002) Oral beclometasone dipropionate in the treatment of active ulcerative colitis: a double-blind placebo-controlled study. Aliment Pharmacol Ther 16(6):1109–1116
20. Campieri M, Adamo S, Valpiani D et al (2003) Oral beclometasone dipropionate in the treatment of extensive and left-sided active ulcerative colitis: a multicentre randomised study. Aliment Pharmacol Ther 17(12):1471–1480
21. Gionchetti P, D'Arienzo A, Rizzello F et al; Italian BDP Study Group (2005) Topical treatment of distal active ulcerative colitis with beclomethasone dipropionate or mesalamine: a single-blind randomized controlled trial. J Clin Gastroenterol 39(4):291–297
22. Biancone L, Gionchetti P, Del Vecchio Blanco G et al (2007) Beclomethasone dipropionate versus mesalazine in distal ulcerative colitis: a multicenter, randomized, double-blind study. Dig Liver Dis 39(4):329–337
23. Campieri M, Cottone M, Miglio F et al (1998) Beclomethasone dipropionate enemas versus prednisolone sodium phosphate enemas in the treatment of distal ulcerative colitis. Aliment Pharmacol Ther 12(4):361–366
24. Bar-Meir S, Fidder HH, Faszczyk M et al; International Budesonide Study Group (2003) Budesonide foam vs. hydrocortisone acetate foam in the treatment of active ulcerative proctosigmoiditis. Dis Colon Rectum 46(7):929–936

25. Gross V, Bar-Meir S, Lavy A et al; International Budesonide Foam Study Group (2006) Budesonide foam versus budesonide enema in active ulcerative proctitis and proctosigmoiditis. Aliment Pharmacol Ther 23(2):303–312

26. Hartmann F, Stein J; BudMesa-Study Group (2010) Clinical trial: controlled, open, randomized multicentre study comparing the effects of treatment on quality of life, safety and efficacy of budesonide or mesalazine enemas in active left-sided ulcerative colitis. Aliment Pharmacol Ther 32(3):368–376

27. Mulder CJ, Fockens P, Meijer JW et al (1996) Beclomethasone dipropionate (3 mg) versus 5-aminosalicylic acid (2 g) versus the combination of both (3 mg/2 g) as retention enemas in active ulcerative proctitis. Eur J Gastroenterol Hepatol 8(6):549–553

28. Marshall JK, Thabane M, Steinhart AH et al (2010) Rectal 5-aminosalicylic acid for induction of remission in ulcerative colitis. Cochrane Database Syst Rev 2010(1):CD004115

29. Gionchetti P, Rizzello F, Venturi A et al (1998) Comparison of oral with rectal mesalazine in the treatment of ulcerative proctitis. Dis Colon Rectum 41(1):93–97

30. van Bodegraven AA, Boer RO, Lourens J et al (1996) Distribution of mesalazine enemas in active and quiescent ulcerative colitis. Aliment Pharmacol Ther 10(3):327–332

31. Andus T, Kocjan A, Müser M et al; International Salofalk Suppository OD Study Group (2010) Clinical trial: a novel high-dose 1 g mesalamine suppository (Salofalk) once daily is as efficacious as a 500-mg suppository thrice daily in active ulcerative proctitis. Inflamm Bowel Dis 16(11):1947–1956

32. Marshall JK, Irvine EJ (1997) Rectal corticosteroids versus alternative treatments in ulcerative colitis: a meta-analysis. Gut 40(6):775–781

33. Ford AC, Khan KJ, Achkar JP; Moayyedi P (2012) Efficacy of oral vs. topical, or combined oral and topical 5-aminosalicylates, in ulcerative colitis: systematic review and meta-analysis. Am J Gastroenterol 107(2):167–176

34. Harbord M, Eliakim R, Bettenworth D et al; European Crohn's and Colitis Organisation [ECCO] (2017) Third European evidence-based consensus on diagnosis and management of ulcerative colitis. Part 2: Current management. J Crohns Colitis 11(7):769–784

35. Ford AC, Achkar J-P, Khan KJ et al (2011) Efficacy of 5-aminosalicylates in ulcerative colitis: systematic review and meta-analysis. Am J Gastroenterol 106(4):601–616

36. Manguso F, Balzano A (2007) Meta-analysis: the efficacy of rectal beclomethasone dipropionate vs. 5-aminosalicylic acid in mild to moderate distal ulcerative colitis. Aliment Pharmacol Ther 26(1):21–29

37. Campieri M, Gionchetti P, Belluzzi A et al (1991) Optimum dosage of 5-aminosalicylic acid as rectal enemas in patients with active ulcerative colitis. Gut 32(8):929–931

38. Wang Y, Parker CE, Bhanji T et al (2016) Oral 5-aminosalicylic acid for induction of remission in ulcerative colitis. Cochrane Database Syst Rev 2016(4):CD000543

39. Feagan BG, MacDonald JK (2012) Once daily oral mesalamine compared to conventional dosing for induction and maintenance of remission in ulcerative colitis: a systematic review and meta-analysis. Inflamm Bowel Dis 18(9):1785–1794

40. Flourié B, Hagège H, Tucat G et al; MOTUS study investigators (2013) Randomised clinical trial: once- vs. twice-daily prolonged-release mesalazine for active ulcerative colitis. Aliment Pharmacol Ther 37(8):767–775

41. Kamm MA, Sandborn WJ, Gassull M et al (2007) Once-daily, high-concentration MMX mesalamine in active ulcerative colitis. Gastroenterology 132(1):66–75

42. Lichtenstein GR, Kamm MA, Boddu P et al (2007) Effect of once- or twice-daily MMX mesalamine (SPD476) for the induction of remission of mild to moderately active ulcerative colitis. Clin Gastroenterol Hepatol 5(1):95–102

43. Sherlock ME, Seow CH, Steinhart AH, Griffiths AM (2010) Oral budesonide for induction of remission in ulcerative colitis. Cochrane Database Syst Rev (10):CD007698

44. Sandborn WJ, Travis S, Moro L et al (2012) Once-daily budesonide MMX extended-release tablets induce remission in patients with mild to moderate ulcerative colitis: results from the CORE I study. Gastroenterology 143(5):1218–1226

45. Travis SP, Danese S, Kupcinskas L et al (2014) Once-daily budesonide MMX in active, mild-to-moderate ulcerative colitis: results from the randomised CORE II study. Gut 63(3):433–441
46. Rubin DT, Cohen RD, Sandborn WJ et al (2017) Budesonide multimatrix is efficacious for mesalamine-refractory, mild to moderate ulcerative colitis: a randomized, placebo-controlled trial. J Crohns Colitis 11(7):785–791
47. Lennard-Jones JE, Longmore AJ, Newell AC et al (1960) An assessment of prednisone, salazopyrin, and topical hydrocortisone hemisuccinate used as out-patient treatment for ulcerative colitis. Gut 1:217–222
48. Truelove SC, Watkinson G, Draper G (1962) Comparison of corticosteroid and sulphasalazine therapy in ulcerative colitis. Br Med J 2(5321):1708–1711
49. Baron JH, Connell AM, Kanaghinis TG et al (1962) Out-patient treatment of ulcerative colitis. Comparison between three doses of oral prednisone. Br Med J 2(5302):441–443
50. Truelove SC, Jewell DP (1974) Intensive intravenous regimen for severe attacks of ulcerative colitis. Lancet 1(7866):106–1070
51. Bossa F, Fiorella S, Caruso N et al (2007) Continuous infusion versus bolus administration of steroids in severe attacks of ulcerative colitis: a randomized, double-blind trial. Am J Gastroenterol 102(3):601–608
52. Turner D, Walsh CM, Steinhart AH, Griffiths AM (2007) Response to corticosteroids in severe ulcerative colitis: a systematic review of the literature and a meta-regression. Clin Gastroenterol Hepatol 5(1):103–110
53. McIntyre PB, Powell-Tuck J, Wood SR et al (1986) Controlled trial of bowel rest in the treatment of severe acute colitis. Gut 27(5):481–485
54. González-Huix F, Fernández-Bañares F, Esteve-Comas M et al (1993) Enteral versus parenteral nutrition as adjunct therapy in acute ulcerative colitis. Am J Gastroenterol 88(2):227–232
55. Chapman RW, Selby WS, Jewell DP (1986) Controlled trial of intravenous metronidazole as an adjunct to corticosteroids in severe ulcerative colitis. Gut 27(10):1210–1212
56. Mantzaris GJ, Hatzis A, Kontogiannis P, Triadaphyllou G (1994) Intravenous tobramycin and metronidazole as an adjunct to corticosteroids in acute, severe ulcerative colitis. Am J Gastroenterol 89(1):43–46
57. Mantzaris GJ, Petraki K, Archavlis E et al (2001) A prospective randomized controlled trial of intravenous ciprofloxacin as an adjunct to corticosteroids in acute, severe ulcerative colitis. Scand J Gastroenterol 36(9):971–974
58. Nguyen GC, Bernstein CN, Bitton A et al (2014) Consensus statements on the risk, prevention, and treatment of venous thromboembolism in inflammatory bowel disease: Canadian Association of Gastroenterology. Gastroenterology 146(3):835–848
59. Travis SP, Farrant JM, Ricketts C et al (1996) Predicting outcome in severe ulcerative colitis. Gut 38(6):905–910
60. Lichtiger S, Present DH, Kornbluth A et al (1994) Cyclosporine in severe ulcerative colitis refractory to steroid therapy. N Engl J Med 330(26):1841–1845
61. Van Assche G, D'Haens G, Noman M et al (2003) Randomized, double-blind comparison of 4 mg/kg versus 2 mg/kg intravenous cyclosporine in severe ulcerative colitis. Gastroenterology 125(4):1025–1031
62. D'Haens G, Lemmens L, Geboes K et al (2001) Intravenous cyclosporine versus intravenous corticosteroids as single therapy for severe attacks of ulcerative colitis. Gastroenterology 120(6):1323–1329
63. Cohen RD, Stein R, Hanauer SB (1999) Intravenous cyclosporin in ulcerative colitis: a five-year experience. Am J Gastroenterol 94(6):1587–1592
64. Moskovitz DN, Van Assche AG, Maenhout B et al (2006) Incidence of colectomy during long-term follow-up after cyclosporine-induced remission of severe ulcerative colitis. Clin Gastroenterol Hepatol 4(6):760–765
65. Shibolet O, Regushevskaya E, Brezis M, Soares-Weiser K (2005) Cyclosporine A for induction of remission in severe ulcerative colitis. Cochrane Database Syst Rev 2005(1):CD004277

66. Fernández-Bañares F, Bertrán X, Esteve-Comas M et al (1996) Azathioprine is useful in maintaining long-term remission induced by intravenous cyclosporine in steroid-refractory severe ulcerative colitis. Am J Gastroenterol 91(12):2498–2499

67. Järnerot G, Hertervig E, Friis-Liby I et al (2005) Infliximab as rescue therapy in severe to moderately severe ulcerative colitis: a randomized, placebo-controlled study. Gastroenterology 128(7):1805–1811

68. Monterubbianesi R, Aratari A, Armuzzi A et al; Italian Group for the study of Inflammatory Bowel Disease (IG-IBD) (2014) Infliximab three-dose induction regimen in severe corticosteroid-refractory ulcerative colitis: early and late outcome and predictors of colectomy. J Crohns Colitis 8(8):852–858

69. Gibson DJ, Heetun ZS, Redmond CE et al (2015) An accelerated infliximab induction regimen reduces the need for early colectomy in patients with acute severe ulcerative colitis. Clin Gastroenterol Hepatol 13(2):330–335

70. Laharie D, Bourreille A, Branche A et al; Groupe d'Etudes Thérapeutiques des Affections Inflammatoires Digestives (2012) Ciclosporin versus infliximab in patients with severe ulcerative colitis refractory to intravenous steroids: a parallel, open-label randomised controlled trial. Lancet 380(9857):1909–1915

71. Williams JG, Alam MF, Alrubaiy L et al (2016) Infliximab versus ciclosporin for steroid-resistant acute severe ulcerative colitis (CONSTRUCT): a mixed methods, open-label, pragmatic randomised trial. Lancet Gastroenterol Hepatol 1(1):15–24

72. Narula N, Fine M, Colombel JF et al (2015) Systematic review: sequential rescue therapy in severe ulcerative colitis: do the benefits outweigh the risks? Inflamm Bowel Dis 21(7):1683–1694

73. Protic M, Seibold F, Schoepfer A et al (2014) The effectiveness and safety of rescue treatments in 108 patients with steroid-refractory ulcerative colitis with sequential rescue therapies in a subgroup of patients. J Crohns Colitis 8(11):1427–1437

74. Gionchetti P, Rizzello F (2014) IBD. Sequential rescue therapy in steroid-refractory ulcerative colitis. Nat Rev Gastroenterol Hepatol 11(9):521–523

75. Hawthorne AB, Logan RF, Hawkey CJ et al (1992) Randomised controlled trial of azathioprine withdrawal in ulcerative colitis. BMJ 305(6844):20–22

76. Jewell DP, Truelove SC (1974) Azathioprine in ulcerative colitis: final report on controlled therapeutic trial. Br Med J 4(5945):627–630

77. Sood A, Kaushal V, Midha V et al (2002) The beneficial effect of azathioprine on maintenance of remission in severe ulcerative colitis. J Gastroenterol 37(4):270–274

78. Maté-Jiménez J, Hermida C, Cantero-Perona J, Moreno-Otero R (2000) 6-mercaptopurine or methotrexate added to prednisone induces and maintains remission in steroid-dependent inflammatory bowel disease. Eur J Gastroenterol Hepatol 12(11):1227–1233

79. Taxonera C, Barreiro-de Acosta M, Calvo M et al (2015) Infliximab dose escalation as an effective strategy for managing secondary loss of response in ulcerative colitis. Dig Dis Sci 60(10):3075–3084

80. Taxonera C, Iglesias E, Muñoz F et al (2017) Adalimumab maintenance treatment in ulcerative colitis: outcomes by prior anti-TNF use and efficacy of dose escalation. Dig Dis Sci 62(2):481–490

81. Armuzzi A, Gionchetti P, Daperno M et al; GIVI (Gruppo Italiano su Vedolizumab nelle IBD) Group (2016) Expert consensus paper on the use of vedolizumab for the management of patients with moderate-to-severe inflammatory bowel disease. Dig Liver Dis 48(4):360–370

Evolution of Surgical Treatment of Ulcerative Colitis

7

Gilberto Poggioli, Lorenzo Gentilini, Maurizio Coscia,
Luca Boschi, and Federica Ugolini

7.1 Introduction

The surgical treatment of ulcerative colitis has changed over time. The aim
of surgical therapy is to completely remove the diseased mucosa with as little
alteration of the normal physiological functions and lifestyle as possible. Four
surgical options have been proposed for patients over time. Initially, all patients
were treated with proctocolectomy and Brooke ileostomy. Subsequently, different surgical options were introduced in order to reduce the disadvantages of a
conventional permanent ileostomy. The main surgical procedures were proctocolectomy and a Kock pouch, abdominal colectomy and ileorectal anastomosis
and, finally, restorative proctocolectomy with ileoanal anastomosis. This last
procedure has become the gold standard of the surgical treatment of ulcerative
colitis; the original technique has also changed over time according to surgical
technical evolutions.

7.2 Proctocolectomy with Brooke Ileostomy

Before 1960, the surgical treatment proposed for all patients with ulcerative
colitis was proctocolectomy with a Brooke ileostomy. This procedure involved
the complete removal of the diseased mucosa of the colon, rectum and anal
canal with the creation of a terminal ileostomy. This approach ensured healing
of patients with, however, the disadvantage of a permanent ileostomy which

L. Gentilini (✉)
General Surgery Unit, Department of Digestive Diseases, S. Orsola-Malpighi Hospital
Bologna, Italy
e-mail: lorenzo.gentilini@aosp.bo.it

G. Poggioli (Ed), *Ulcerative Colitis,*
Updates in Surgery
DOI: 10.1007/978-88-470-3977-3_7, © Springer-Verlag Italia 2019

could negatively influence quality of life (QoL), especially social and sexual functions. Moreover, there were many postoperative complications related to this procedure. Sexual function could be impaired by erectile and ejaculation dysfunctions due to nerve injuries which can occur during the pelvic dissection associated with the proctectomy. Moreover, several patients reported a delay in perineal wound healing, with the development of postoperative chronic perineal sinus accompanied by subsequent disabling leakage. Proctocolectomy with Brooke ileostomy has been replaced over time by surgical procedures which ensure the preservation of transanal defecation. Currently, this procedure can be offered to patients who have already undergone restorative proctocolectomy with ileoanal anastomosis but who have reported pouch failure. A primary proctectomy with Brooke ileostomy should also be reserved for patients who wish to avoid the problems associated with an ileoanal pouch procedure, such as long-term pouch complications and poor pouch function, for patients with poor sphincter function due to previous surgery, or in the elderly.

7.3   Proctocolectomy with the Kock Pouch

This procedure was introduced in Göteborg in 1969 by Professor Nils Kock. The Kock pouch procedure involved a standard proctocolectomy with creation of an ileal pouch prior to the ileostomy having a valve to render the ileostomy continent. It was initially proposed by Kock as a continent urinary pouch in cats and was subsequently applied as a continent ileostomy in humans. Approximately 50 cm of the small bowel were utilized for the procedure. The distal most 3–5 cm were used for the outlet, the following 18 cm proximal to this were utilized for construction of the nipple valve and approximately 30 cm were used for the Kock pouch, which had originally been proposed as a U- or an S-pouch. The valve is created by intussusception of the terminal ileum into the pouch, with prior stripping of the mesentery and fat over the ileum, which is to be made into the nipple valve [1].

The pouch is emptied by tube intubation two to four times daily. An external appliance is not needed.

In the early 1970s, multiple authors described good functional outcomes in patients undergoing a Kock pouch procedure [2]. The indications at that time were specifically for patients not wishing to have a conventional ileostomy, as this was an alternative to total proctocolectomy and ileostomy. It provided the patient with a mechanism for continence and overcame a significant number of the psychosocial problems related to a conventional ileostomy. However, the procedure itself was, and still is, a complex one, with numerous complications. In the first years after surgery, the reoperation rate reached up to 35% of patients in experienced centers and was much higher in centers with limited experience.

The most common problem is nipple valve dysfunction. The valve can become inherently unstable with subsequent difficulties with intubation or incontinence of the pouch. Valve necrosis can occur early following construction of the pouch, due to ischemia resulting from excision of the peritoneum and fat from the mesentery of the segment of ileum forming the valve, or the placement of staples across the mesentery reducing blood supply to the valve. Fistulas occur in 8–12% of patients while pouchitis is a frequent condition occurring in 8–42% of patients.

Today, the main indication for a Kock pouch is in those patients seeking an alternative to a conventional ileostomy owing to skin problems, psychosocial and sexual problems, or failed ileoanal pouch procedures. It could also be suggested for patients who have previously undergone a proctocolectomy and Brooke ileostomy and who wish conversion due to dissatisfaction with the ileostomy [3].

7.4 Abdominal Colectomy and Ileorectal Anastomosis

Between 1960 and 1980 abdominal colectomy and ileorectal anastomosis (IRA) was proposed as an alternative option to proctocolectomy with the Kock pouch procedure. This operation involved removal of the abdominal colon with creation of an ileorectal anastomosis, leaving the diseased rectum in situ with a simple sphincter-saving operation. It was proposed for patients who wished to avoid a permanent stoma. This single stage operation was associated with minimum hospital stay and low rates of complications, and with significant reduction in bladder and sexual dysfunction secondary to pelvic nerve injury [4, 5]. The rectum should be transected at the level of the sacral promontory, and not mobilized, so as to avoid damage to the nervi erigentes while descending over the edge of the pelvis and passing down to the inferior hypogastric plexus.

In a recent retrospective study, 22 IRA patients were compared to 66 ileal pouch-anal anastomosis (IPAA) patients, showing that the first group had a significantly lower defecation frequency per day and less night-time seepage, but greater urgency, and more dietary and work restrictions than the second group; the QoL was similar in both groups [5].

Although the QoL after surgery was generally satisfactory, many patients required chronic maintenance therapy to treat residual proctitis. Moreover, the functional results were significantly influenced by rectal compliance, and by the extension and activity of the ulcerative colitis. Good functional results have been obtained in approximately 80–90% of carefully selected patients, having an average of 4–5 stools per 24 hours and nocturnal evacuation occurring in approximately 35% of patients.

This operation should not be undertaken in patients with active rectal disease or in those with colonic or rectal dysplasia. An ileorectal anastomosis in patients with an inflamed rectum is associated with a higher number of bowel movements and a higher rate of incontinence.

Regarding the long-term results, many authors have emphasized the disadvantages of IRA due to the preservation of the rectum, with the risk of developing intractable proctitis or cancer in the rectal stump [6–8]. Many patients required a subsequent proctectomy due to the severe recurrence of proctitis or to malignant degeneration. The most important long-term complication was the development of rectal cancer. It has been reported that, after IRA, there was a risk of rectal cancer which increased with the time elapsed after surgery [8]. The risk of malignant degeneration was 5–6% at 20 years, 15% at 30 years and 18% at 35 years; therefore, patients required careful endoscopic surveillance. For this reason, the cumulative probability of having a functional ileorectal anastomosis has decreased significantly over time; only 50% of patients had a still functioning ileorectal anastomosis 10 years after surgery, and this probability decreased to 32% 20 years since colectomy [8].

7.5   Restorative Proctocolectomy with Ileoanal Anastomosis

Restorative proctocolectomy was first described by Sir Alan Parks and Nicholls of St Mark's Hospital in London in 1978 and it is currently the procedure of choice for the surgical treatment of patients with ulcerative colitis [9]. Parks and Nicholls combined elements of Kock's continent pouch with a technique of rectal mucosal excision developed for the removal of rectal adenomas and hemangiomas. The ileal pouch reservoir was anastomosed to the dentate line using a per-anal suturing technique. This procedure allowed the complete removal of the diseased mucosa with healing of the patient, thus avoiding a permanent stoma. The initial results were sufficiently positive to lead to additional studies; the effectiveness of the procedure – as demonstrated by measurements of patient function, QoL parameters, and the enthusiasm of surgeons and gastroenterologists – has led to its widespread adoption by the colorectal surgical community. In a relatively short period of time, this technique has become the preferred surgical option for the treatment of ulcerative colitis. However, since its introduction, the operation has undergone multiple modifications due to the evolution of surgical techniques. Changes to the original technique have been carried out in order to reduce surgical time and to make the procedure simpler; moreover, several changes in surgical technique have led to improvement in the functional results.

Parks and Nicholls initially proposed a hand-sewn pouch with an "S" configuration [9]. The S-pouch was created using 3 limbs of 12 to 15 cm of terminal small bowel, hand-sutured together, with a 3 cm exit conduit which was hand-sutured to the anal canal. Before performing the anastomosis, patients underwent mucosectomy. Initially, the retained rectal muscular cuff was left at 8–10 cm as in the Soave procedure (long mucosectomy). With evolution of the technique, a short mucosectomy was introduced; currently, only 1–2 cm of retained rectal cuff are left in situ, significantly reducing the incidence of pelvic intramuscular cuff abscess.

The length of the efferent limb of the S-pouch has also been reduced over time due to problems in bowel evacuation. In fact, many patients treated with this procedure reported evacuation problems leading to the need for pouch intubation in up to 50% of cases [10]. To reduce the incidence of evacuation problems, the 3 cm efferent limb has been shortened to 1–2 cm, with subsequent improvement in pouch function.

The technical difficulty of the original S-pouch construction motivated the development of less complex alternatives; the J-pouch was described by Utsunomiya in 1980 [11], and then the 4-limbed W-pouch was described by Nicholls et al. in 1985 [10]. Subsequently, other designs of pouches, such as K [12], H [13], B [14], and U [15] have been proposed. However, those were not completely validated by subsequent studies and did not reach wide diffusion in clinical practice. The J pouch introduced by Utsunomiya was constructed using 30 to 40 cm of terminal ileum. This segment of ileum was folded into two 15 or 20 cm segments which were sutured together side to side. The first advantage of this procedure as compared to the S-pouch was that it could be performed using staplers, significantly reducing operative time. Originally this pouch was proposed 15 cm in length, but its dimension was subsequently increased up to 20 cm. However, higher dimensions have been associated with pouch retention and difficulty in emptying. Currently, a J-pouch ranges from 15–18 cm and is tailored to patient size.

The W-pouch was proposed by Nicholls and Pezim in 1985 [10]. They introduced the design of this pouch because of the potential advantages of lower frequency of defecation and no requirement for pouch intubation. Similar to the S-pouch, the W-pouch must also be hand-sewn, using approximately 50 cm of terminal ileum. This design combined the advantages of both the J-and the S-pouch; however, it was technically more difficult to construct and more time-consuming. Moreover, its bulkiness could also result in greater difficulties in placing the pouch into a narrow pelvis.

The evidence demonstrates that, in the short term, within the first year of pouch function, its performance is related to volume and compliance and, consequently, appears to be better with the W- or even the S-pouch design. Patients with S- or W-pouches report a lower number of bowel movements and lesser use of antimotility drugs when compared to patients with J-pouches. However, as the pouch matures, the functional disparity between the pouches lessens or even disappears. According to these data, the J-pouch is actually the most widespread in the world due to the technical feasibility associated with satisfactory functional outcomes. The S-pouch is actually preferred when a J-pouch does not reach into the pelvis without tension and lengthening of the ileum is not possible or not sufficient.

Another technical evolution has been represented by the introduction of stapled anastomosis. The advent of stapling instruments greatly simplified ileal pouch-anal anastomosis surgery. Stapling was first described by Johnston in 1987 who proposed an end-to-end ileoanal anastomosis without mucosal resection using an endo-anal stapled anastomosis [16]. Since the introduction of this technique, restorative proctocolectomy has become faster and easier; moreover, when using this approach, the anal transition zone was preserved, resulting in better functional outcomes due to preservation of the rich sensory innervations present in this zone and involved in differentiating between flatus and stool. Moreover, with a stapled anastomosis, the manipulation of the anal canal was also reduced, therefore decreasing the risk of postoperative problems with continence.

Several studies have analyzed long-term functional outcomes in patients undergoing both hand-sewn and stapled anastomoses. The data obtained have shown a superiority of stapled anastomosis in terms of functional outcomes. Patients treated with this approach have reported a lower rate of seepage at night and incontinence of liquid stool with subsequent reduced use of protective pads during the night; dietary, social and work restrictions were also lower in these patients [17, 18]. No differences have been reported over time between these two techniques of anastomosis regarding both pouch failure and the incidence of postoperative complications, such as anastomotic leak, pelvic sepsis, pouch-related fistula, pouchitis and anastomotic stricture, thus showing that the technique was effective and safe [17, 18].

Therefore, currently a stapled IPAA is the preferred technique because it is easier and quicker to perform, and is associated with better long-term functional outcomes. A hand-sewn anastomosis is preferred in patients having a failure of the stapled technique or in patients requiring redo surgery. Total proctocolectomy and IPAA can be performed in one, two or three stages [19]:

- *1-stage procedure*: total proctocolectomy, ileal pouch construction and IPAA are performed during the same surgery without ileostomy;
- *2-stage procedure*: total proctocolectomy, ileal pouch construction and IPAA are performed during the same surgery with a diverting ileostomy; 3 months after the first stage, patients undergo ileostomy reversal;
- *2-stage-modified procedure*: the first stage is a subtotal colectomy with closure of the rectal stump and its suture to the subcutaneous tissue as a mucous fistula (in order to avoid rectal stump breakdown and leakage with subsequent pelvic sepsis, especially in the case of severe proctitis); 6–8 months after the first stage, patients are scheduled for proctectomy, pouch construction and IPAA without ileostomy;

- *3-stage procedure*: the first stage is a subtotal colectomy with the creation of end ileostomy closure of the rectal stump; 6-8 months after the first stage, patients undergo proctectomy, pouch construction and IPAA with diverting loop ileostomy; 3 months after the second stage, the patients undergo ileostomy reversal.

The initial expectation of the surgeons was to use a multiple-stage procedure to perform a restorative proctocolectomy with IPAA; this initial approach has been modified over time to increase the use of single-stage surgical strategy. This tendency has again been reversed in the last decade towards an increased use of 3-stage procedures, perhaps due to changes in preoperative medical therapy [20, 21].

7.6   Minimally Invasive Surgery

Similar to colorectal surgery, the surgical treatment of ulcerative colitis also changed with the introduction of the laparoscopic approach. Many studies have reported the importance of minimally invasive techniques in patients with inflammatory bowel disease. These studies showed that laparoscopic restorative proctocolectomy was feasible and safe without significant differences when compared to an open approach in terms of early and late postoperative complications or pouch retention rate. Similar to colorectal surgery, laparoscopic surgery in patients with ulcerative colitis was associated with enhanced postoperative recovery, fastened restoration of intestinal continuity, improved female fecundity, and improved body image and cosmesis [22–24]. A recent meta-analysis has reported similar functional outcomes between laparoscopic and open restorative proctocolectomy [25]. Based on these data, the laparoscopic approach in the treatment of ulcerative colitis has become very popular in the last decade.

However, distal dissection of the rectum is still difficult with a laparoscopic approach and it represents the most challenging step of this surgical procedure. If the section of the rectum is too high, it could lead to the retention of a long rectal cuff which may evolve into cuffitis, fistula formation and poor pouch function. This condition cannot definitively be treated with medical therapy and frequently requires salvage surgery.

To overcome the technical hurdles occurring during laparoscopic pelvic dissection and distal rectal transection modern technologies have arisen to assist the surgeon. Transanal ileal pouch-anal anastomosis (ta-IPAA) has been proposed for patients with ulcerative colitis. In addition to better pelvic accessibility, transanal access gives the surgeon the opportunity of more appropriately deciding on the level of the anastomosis at the top of the transition zone. A recent study published in 2017 showed that ta-IPAA was safe, with decreasing rates of postoperative morbidity. Moreover, it had a favorable impact on the occurrence of delayed resumption of oral intake and postoperative length of hospital stay, without any significant impact on the duration of surgery. Surgeons using the transanal approach had a significantly lower conversion rate without differences in the incidence of anastomotic leakage [26].

7.7   Salvage Surgery after Failed Restorative Proctocolectomy

Restorative proctocolectomy is one of the most important advances in colorectal surgery in the past 50 years. It has allowed thousands of patients to avoid a permanent ileostomy and to live relatively normal lives free from continued medication, the risk of cancer linked to colitis and polyposis. However, currently, some 5–10% of IPAA procedures fail [27]. Three-quarters of the pouches failed because of sepsis or obstruction. Pelvic sepsis can be associated with anastomotic leaks or pouch fistulas. If sepsis occurs after the fashioning of an ileoanal pouch, early and adequate treatment may prevent chronic sepsis and pouch failure. Other possible causes of pouch failure are chronic ischemia due to twists in the pouch mesentery, a delayed diagnosis of Crohn's disease with subsequent inflammation of the body of the pouch or fistula formation, retention of a long rectal stump which could lead to the onset of severe cuffitis or the onset of inflammatory complications, such as severe chronic pouchitis or pre-pouch ileitis. The evolution in pouch surgery has allowed the introduction of new procedures for the salvage surgery of the pouch. Salvage surgery procedures are demanding procedures which should be performed only in highly selected centers. Redo-surgery includes redo-pouch, redo-anastomosis or remodeling of the pouch itself. With a redo-pouch procedure, the failed pouch should be removed and a new pouch should be fashioned. In many cases, the new pouch could have difficulties in reaching the pelvic floor without tension so a hand-sewn anastomosis with good lengthening of the ileum is suggested. In the presence of excessive tension, an S-pouch will reach further into the pelvis than a J-pouch owing to the presence of a long efferent limb; therefore, it is preferred. A redo-anastomosis is recommended in patients with a long rectal stump or severe cuffitis; this procedure allows preserving the original pouch, fashioning a new pouch-anal anastomosis. The new anastomosis is usually hand-sewn, performed after the removal of the rectal stump. In patients who report poor pouch function not related to septic complications but due to the wide volume of the pouch, salvage surgery can be performed by resizing the pouch itself without resection. Since its introduction, redo pouch surgery has improved over time. Currently, approximately three-fourths of patients undergoing redo-surgery now retain a functional pouch in the long term [28].

Salvage surgery is still associated with a high rate of postoperative complications. Complications arising as a result of redo IPAA occurred in 46% of patients.

These results indicate that, even in the best hands, redo surgery carries an appreciable morbidity rate. The main postoperative complications are septic; patients who developed a recurrent pelvic sepsis after redo ileal pouch surgery are at risk for failure of their revised pouch. Not surprisingly, outcomes are worse in terms of both overall failure and function when compared with first-time surgery; nevertheless, this procedure remains a valid alternative to a defunctioning stoma or pouch excision.

Several studies have analyzed functional outcomes and QoL in patients undergoing salvage surgery concluding that these procedures were associated with acceptable long-term functional results. After redo surgery, patients have reported high rates of incontinence and seepage with the subsequent increased use of protective pads. Despite this, patients stated an almost universal willingness to have the surgery again if it were necessary and to recommend the surgery to others. This is likely to reflect more their dread of a permanent ileostomy than their happiness with their continence and bowel habits [29, 30].

Therefore, redo pouch surgery can finally allow good outcomes in the majority patients, although it is at high risk of postoperative complications; for this reason, salvage surgery should be proposed only to highly motivated patients.

References

1. Cranley B (1983) The Kock reservoir ileostomy: a review of its development, problems and role in modern surgical practice. Br J Surg 70(2):94–99
2. Fazio VW, Church JM (1988) Complications and function of the continent ileostomy at the Cleveland Clinic. World J Surg 12(2):148–154
3. Schrock TR (1979) Complications of continent ileostomy. Am J Surg 138(1):162–169
4. Börjesson L, Lundstam U, Øresland T et al (2006) The place for colectomy and ileorectal anastomosis: a valid surgical option for ulcerative colitis? Tech Coloproctol 10(3):237–241
5. da Luz Moreira A, Kiran RP, Lavery I (2010) Clinical outcomes of ileorectal anastomosis for ulcerative colitis. Br J Surg 97(1):65–69
6. Leijonmarck CE, Löfberg R, Ost A, Hellers G (1990) Long-term results of ileorectal anastomosis in ulcerative colitis in Stockholm County. Dis Colon Rectum 33(3):195–200
7. Baker WN, Glass RE, Ritchie JK, Aylett SO (1978) Cancer of the rectum following colectomy and ileorectal anastomosis for ulcerative colitis. Br J Surg 65(12):862–868
8. Böhm G, O'Dwyer ST (2007) The fate of the rectal stump after subtotal colectomy for ulcerative colitis. Int J Colorectal Dis 22(3):277–282
9. Parks AG, Nicholls RJ (1978) Proctocolectomy without ileostomy for ulcerative colitis. Br Med J 2(6130):85–88
10. Nicholls RJ, Pezim ME (1985) Restorative proctocolectomy with ileal reservoir for ulcerative colitis and familial adenomatous polyposis: a comparison of three reservoir designs. Br J Surg 72(6):470–474
11. Utsunomiya J, Iwama T, Imajo M et al (1980) Total colectomy, mucosal proctectomy, and ileoanal anastomosis. Dis Colon Rectum 23(7):459–466
12. Hallgren T, Fasth S, Nordgren S et al (1989) Manovolumetric characteristics and functional results in three different pelvic pouch designs. Int J Colorectal Dis 4(3):156–160
13. Fonkalsrud EW (1987) Update on clinical experience with different surgical techniques of the endorectal pull-through operation for colitis and polyposis. Surg Gynecol Obstet 165(4):309–316

14. Slors JF, Taat CW, Brummelkamp WH (1989) Ileal pouch-anal anastomosis without rectal muscular cuff. Int J Colorectal Dis 4(3):178–181
15. Nelson RL, Prasad LM, Pearl RK, Abcarian H (1991) Inverted U-pouch construction for restoration of function in patients with failed straight ileoanal pull-throughs. Dis Colon Rectum 34(11):1040–1042
16. Johnston D, Holdsworth PJ, Nasmyth DG et al (1987) Preservation of the entire anal canal in conservative proctocolectomy for ulcerative colitis: a pilot study comparing end-to-end ileo-anal anastomosis without mucosal resection with mucosal proctectomy and endo-anal anastomosis. Br J Surg 74(10):940–944
17. Lovegrove RE, Constantinides VA, Heriot AG et al (2006) A comparison of hand-sewn versus stapled ileal pouch anal anastomosis (IPAA) following proctocolectomy: a meta-analysis of 4183 patients. Ann Surg 244(1):18–26
18. Kirat HT, Remzi FH, Kiran RP, Fazio VW (2009) Comparison of outcomes after hand-sewn versus stapled ileal pouch-anal anastomosis in 3,109 patients. Surgery 146(4):723–729; discussion 729–730
19. Melville DM, Ritchie JK, Nicholls RJ, Hawley PR (1994) Surgery for ulcerative colitis in the era of the pouch: the St Mark's Hospital experience. Gut 35(8):1076–1080
20. Zittan E, Wong-Chong N, Ma GW et al (2016) Modified two-stage ileal pouch-anal anastomosis results in lower rate of anastomotic leak compared with traditional two-stage surgery for ulcerative colitis. J Crohns Colitis 10(7):766–772
21. Swenson BR, Hollenbeak CS, Poritz LS, Koltun WA (2005) Modified two-stage ileal pouch-anal anastomosis: equivalent outcomes with less resource utilization. Dis Colon Rectum 48(2):256–261
22. Bartels SA, Gardenbroek TJ, Ubbink DT et al (2013) Systematic review and meta-analysis of laparoscopic versus open colectomy with end ileostomy for non-toxic colitis. Br J Surg 100(6):726–733
23. Fajardo AD, Dharmarajan S, George V et al (2010) Laparoscopic versus open 2-stage ileal pouch: laparoscopic approach allows for faster restoration of intestinal continuity. J Am Coll Surg 211(3):377–383
24. Bartels SA, D'Hoore A, Cuesta MA et al (2012) Significantly increased pregnancy rates after laparoscopic restorative proctocolectomy: a cross-sectional study. Ann Surg 256(6):1045–1048
25. Singh P, Bhangu A, Nicholls RJ, Tekkis P (2013) A systematic review and meta-analysis of laparoscopic vs open restorative proctocolectomy. Colorectal Dis 15(7):e340–e351
26. de Buck van Overstraeten A, Mark-Christensen A, Wasmann KA et al (2017) Transanal versus transabdominal minimally invasive (completion) proctectomy with ileal pouch-anal anastomosis in ulcerative colitis: a comparative study. Ann Surg 266(5):878–883
27. Fazio VW, Kiran RP, Remzi FH et al (2013) Ileal pouch anal anastomosis: analysis of outcome and quality of life in 3707 patients. Ann Surg 257(4):679–685
28. MacLean AR, O'Connor B, Parkes R et al (2002) Reconstructive surgery for failed ileal pouch-anal anastomosis: a viable surgical option with acceptable results. Dis Colon Rectum 45(7):880–886
29. Theodoropoulos GE, Choman EN, Wexner SD (2015) Salvage procedures after restorative proctocolectomy: a systematic review and meta-analysis. J Am Coll Surg 220(2):225–242
30. Remzi FH, Aytac E, Ashburn J et al (2015) Transabdominal redo ileal pouch surgery for failed restorative proctocolectomy: lessons learned over 500 patients. Ann Surg 262(4):675–682

Surgical Treatment of Ulcerative Colitis: How Has the Timing of Surgery Changed?

8

Gilberto Poggioli, Laura Vittori, Federico Ghignone, Lorenzo Gentilini, and Maurizio Coscia

8.1   Introduction

Restorative proctocolectomy with ileal pouch-anal anastomosis (IPAA) still represents the surgical cornerstone for the treatment of ulcerative colitis (UC). This surgical technique was developed in the second half of the last century when Ravitch and Sabiston first proposed the creation of a straight ileal anastomosis to the anus following proctocolectomy [1]. In subsequent years, Parks and Nicholls combined the key concepts of Kock's continent pouch with the techniques for rectal mucosa excision of benign lesions, introducing IPAA after proctocolectomy for UC for the first time [2].

In past decades, acute colitis with toxic megacolon was the most frequent presentation in patients affected by UC; an emergency subtotal colectomy with end ileostomy was a life-saving treatment to be followed later by the creation of a pouch under elective conditions. An old retrospective analysis from St. Mark's Hospital in London showed a 25% rate of colectomy in an emergency setting [3]. Nowadays, massive widespread effective medical therapies in clinical practice offer conservative treatments before referring patients to surgeons; currently, only a minority (5–8%) of patients manifest symptoms and signs of acute severe colitis at the time of diagnosis [4] and few of them will require immediate surgery for salvage medical therapy failure. For this reason, indications for surgery have progressively shifted to disease refractoriness due to drug resistance, steroid dependence, growth impairment in children and the onset of dysplasia or cancer.

L. Gentilini (✉)
General Surgery Unit, Department of Digestive Diseases, S. Orsola-Malpighi Hospital
Bologna, Italy
e-mail: lorenzo.gentilini@aosp.bo.it

G. Poggioli (Ed), *Ulcerative Colitis*,
Updates in Surgery
DOI: 10.1007/978-88-470-3977-3_8, © Springer-Verlag Italia 2019

8.2   Surgical Procedure

Ileal pouch-anal anastomosis can be performed in one, two or three stages
(Fig 8.1). The surgical procedure consists of a first demolition phase
(proctocolectomy) and a following reconstructive phase (pouch construction
and pouch-anal anastomosis):
- *1-stage procedure*: total proctocolectomy, ileal pouch construction and IPAA
  are performed during the same surgery without ileostomy;
- *2-stage procedure*: total proctocolectomy, ileal pouch construction and IPAA
  are performed during the same surgery with a diverting loop ileostomy; 3
  months after the first stage, patients undergo ileostomy reversal;
- *2-stage-modified procedure*: the first stage is a subtotal colectomy with
  closure of the rectal stump and its suture to the subcutaneous tissue as a
  mucous fistula (in order to avoid rectal stump breakdown and leakage with
  subsequent pelvic sepsis, especially in the case of severe proctitis); 6–8
  months after the first stage, patients are scheduled for proctectomy, pouch
  construction and IPAA without ileostomy;
- *3-stage procedure*: the first stage is a subtotal colectomy with the creation of
  end ileostomy closure of the rectal stump; 6–8 months after the first stage,
  patients undergo proctectomy, pouch construction and IPAA with diverting
  loop ileostomy; 3 months after the second stage, the patients undergo
  ileostomy reversal.

The choice of the single- or multiple-stage approach is made by the surgeon
and depends on many different factors, such as clinical presentation (i.e., acute
vs. chronic or active vs. remissive colitis), general condition, comorbidities,
nutritional status and pharmacologic history.

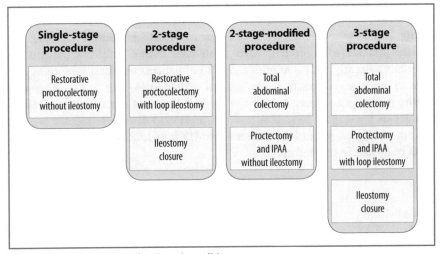

Fig. 8.1 Surgical procedures for ulcerative colitis

The 1-stage procedure is an elective operation usually performed in the absence of toxicity or severe malnutrition. This operation is indicated in healthy, well-nourished and steroid-free patients who are not experiencing acute flares. It could also be indicated in patients with colonic dysplasia or cancer arising from quiescent UC. It was definitely more common in the last two decades of the 20th century and is presently extremely rare owing to the use (or sometimes abuse) of conservative medical treatments.

The incidence and the severity of surgical complications depend on the surgical time considered (1st stage vs 2nd stage) and are more severe when reconstructive surgery is performed. The rationale of the diverting ileostomy is not to prevent pelvic sepsis in the setting of the IPAA, but to lessen complications in the case of anastomotic leakage, lowering the risk of pouch excision/failure and giving surgeons greater opportunities for conservative treatments (i.e., operative endoscopy, percutaneous drainage, etc.).

A staged procedure is recommended in acute colitis or in patients treated with steroids or anti-tumor necrosis factor (TNF). In these settings, a 3-stage procedure is considered safer for patients. The 2-stage-modified approach could be the solution for patients who are not fit for single-stage surgery, at the moment of the surgical indication, but could instead benefit from the post-colectomy phase for the purpose of a wash-out from drugs, gaining adequate body weight and facing up to the restorative surgery under better health conditions. In recent years, together with the widespread diffusion of laparoscopy, several studies have shown a progressive increase in the 2-stage-modified procedure claiming a lower incidence of IPAA-related anastomotic complications and a better quality of life [5–8]. In addition, it is mandatory for surgeons to keep in mind that IPAA surgery is always technically demanding and the results regarding preoperative medical therapy still under debate. For this reason, given the decrease in the number of complications related to ileostomy take-down as compared to IPAA creation, a 3-stage procedure is often to be preferred, as it considered to be safer for patients.

Furthermore, the multistage procedure (starting with a total abdominal colectomy) is suggested for indeterminate colitis and/or for all cases in which Crohn's disease (CD) cannot be excluded. When a subtotal colectomy is first performed, a proper waiting time before proctectomy and IPAA creation is suggested in order to avoid surgical complications after the restorative phase. A delayed second surgery is suggested to allow patients to recover from severely ill clinical conditions, to be weaned from high doses of immunosuppressive drugs and to diminish intra-abdominal adhesions [9]. Various retrospective studies have been focused on the time gap between the different stages of surgery, and a significantly higher rate of intra- and postoperative complications (i.e., anastomotic fistulas) was found in restorative proctectomy performed less than 6–8 months after the primary surgery [10].

8.3   Pharmacological Treatment and Surgery

Medical therapy is effective in many cases but there is clear evidence that a delay in surgery, when indicated, is detrimental for patient outcomes; collaboration between the surgeon and the gastroenterologist is, therefore, mandatory in order to monitor the flare of disease and the timing for surgery.

8.3.1   Steroids

Looking at the pharmacologic history of UC patients who have undergone surgery, it is well known that a long-time history of systemic steroids can increase the risk of anastomotic leakage and subsequent pelvic sepsis. The incidence of surgical complications after restorative proctocolectomy is 3.8%, 20% and 50% in low, medium and high dosage steroidal treatment, respectively [11, 12]. The latest European Crohn's and Colitis Organisation (ECCO) guidelines state that a staged proctocolectomy with subtotal colectomy must be considered in patients who have received prolonged steroid therapy (more than 20 mg of prednisolone/day for longer than 6 weeks). A subtotal colectomy with an ileostomy will spare patients from the burden of colitis. As a consequence, they will regain general health, normalize their diet, and have the time to carefully consider the options of an IPAA or of a permanent ileostomy [13].

8.3.2   Immunosuppressive Therapy

Immunosuppressive therapy seems to be the pharmacological category which plays a minor role in postoperative complications after the restorative stage. It does not increase the incidence of septic complications in patients with a diagnosis of UC, unlike subjects affected by CD (in fact, in this subset of patients the higher risk of complications after surgery has been well documented) [14]. However, a suspension of at least 3 months before surgery is suggested, even in the case of UC.

8.3.3   Biological Therapies

Anti-TNF therapy has become a common medical strategy since its introduction in inflammatory bowel disease (IBD) treatment, with optimal response in patients affected by moderate-severe activity disease with no response to traditional therapy. The introduction of these molecules has drastically changed the behavior of the disease, with a decrease in toxic megacolon and acute colitis. Conversely, the number of patients undergoing surgery for chronic refractory disease has greatly increased.

Since it has clearly been demonstrated that no higher incidence of postoperative complications has been reported after colectomy in UC patients previously treated with biological agents [15], many studies have tried to identify a clear relationship between biological therapy and postoperative complications. The first studies conducted approximately 10 years ago in two international referral centers (the Mayo Clinic and the Cleveland Clinic Foundation) [16, 17], compared postoperative complications after reconstructive surgery (proctectomy, construction of an ileal pouch and pouch-anal anastomosis) in biologic-treated patients versus naïve ones. Both studies demonstrated higher septic postoperative complications in the biological therapy cohort, in particular the early onset of anastomotic leakage and/or pelvic abscess. The higher risk of postoperative anastomotic leak and pelvic sepsis after IPAA can be avoided if patients who undergo biological therapy are candidates for a 3-stage procedure [18] or if the pharmacological therapy is interrupted 12 weeks before surgery [19]. In addition, the ECCO guidelines state "As long as the data on perioperative use of anti-TNF agents remain conflicting, the standing recommendation is to not perform a single stage proctocolectomy with ileo-anal pouch construction in anti-TNF treated patients" [4]. As a consequence, in the last decade an increasing number of 2- or 3-stage procedures has been observed worldwide.

Recently, new biological agents, such as vedolizumab and golimumab, have been introduced into the medical management of UC. The literature regarding the relationship between these molecules and postoperative complications after pouch creation is limited. A retrospective analysis from the Mayo Clinic involving 88 patients previously treated with vedolizumab showed a significantly increased superficial surgical site infection; of the IPAA patients, peri-pouch abscess rates increased in the vedolizumab-treated patients, but this did not reach statistical significance [20]. No data regarding the preoperative use and postoperative complications of golimumab is currently available.

8.4   Conclusion

In conclusion, recent advancements in medical therapy have not reduced surgical need but have just delayed it according to the natural evolution of UC. Prolonged history of or ongoing high dose steroid therapy at the time of surgery represents a major contraindication to a 1- or 2-stage-modified procedure; adequate washout from immunosuppressive drugs is suggested whenever possible, even if no significant data regarding risk for postoperative complications have been reported.

The preoperative use of biologic agents should be considered a risk factor for pouch-related complications (pelvic abscess, anastomotic leakage) in patients selected for restorative proctocolectomy. Preoperative multidisciplinary evaluation should be mandatory in order to plan early withdrawal of the anti-TNF therapy (at least 3 months before surgery); whenever not possible, subtotal colectomy with an end ileostomy should be considered the treatment of choice.

References

1. Ravitch MM, Sabiston DC Jr (1947) Anal ileostomy with preservation of the sphincter; a proposed operation in patients requiring total colectomy for benign lesions. Surg Gynecol Obstet 84(6):1095–1099
2. Parks AG, Nicholls RJ (1978) Proctocolectomy without ileostomy for ulcerative colitis. Br Med J 2(6130):85–88
3. Melville DM, Ritchie JK, Nicholls RJ, Hawley PR (1994) Surgery for ulcerative colitis in the era of the pouch: the St Mark's Hospital experience. Gut 35(8):1076–1080
4. Strong SA (2010) Management of acute colitis and toxic megacolon. Clin Colon Rectal Surg 23(4):274–284
5. Samples J, Evans K, Chaumont N et al (2017) Variant two-stage ileal pouch-anal anastomosis: an innovative and effective alternative to standard resection in ulcerative colitis. J Am Coll Surg 224(4):557–563
6. Zittan E, Wong-Chong N, Ma GW et al (2016) Modified two-stage ileal pouch-anal anastomosis results in lower rate of anastomotic leak compared with traditional two-stage surgery for ulcerative colitis. J Crohns Colitis 10(7):766–772
7. Germain A, de Buck van Overstraeten A, Wolthuis A (2018) Outcome of restorative proctocolectomy with ileo-anal pouch for ulcerative colitis: effect of changes in clinical practice. Colorectal Dis 20(2):O30–O38
8. Swenson BR, Hollenbeak CS, Poritz LS, Koltun WA (2005) Modified two-stage ileal pouch-anal anastomosis: equivalent outcomes with less resource utilization. Dis Colon Rectum 48(2):256–261
9. Spinelli A, Sampietro GM, Bazzi P et al (2011) Surgical approach to ulcerative colitis: when is the best timing after medical treatment? Current Drug Targets 12(10):1462–1466
10. Dinnewitzer AJ, Wexner SD, Baig MK et al (2006) Timing of restorative proctectomy following subtotal colectomy in patients with inflammatory bowel disease. Colorectal Dis 8(4):278–282
11. Ziv Y, Church JM, Fazio VW et al (1996) Effect of systemic steroids on ileal pouch-anal anastomosis in patients with ulcerative colitis. Dis Colon Rectum 39(5):504–508
12. Lake JP, Firoozmand E, Kang JC et al (2004) Effect of high-dose steroids on anastomotic complications after proctocolectomy with ileal pouch-anal anastomosis. J Gastrointest Surg 8(5):547–551
13. Magro F, Gionchetti P, Eliakim R et al; European Crohn's and Colitis Organisation [ECCO] (2017) Third European evidence-based consensus on diagnosis and management of ulcerative colitis. Part 1: definitions, diagnosis, extra-intestinal manifestations, pregnancy, cancer surveillance, surgery, and ileo-anal pouch disorders. J Crohns Colitis 11(6):649–670
14. Mahadevan U, Loftus EV Jr, Tremaine WJ et al (2002) Azathioprine or 6-mercaptopurine before colectomy for ulcerative colitis is not associated with increased postoperative complications. Inflamm Bowel Dis 8(5):311–316
15. Bregnbak D, Mortensen C, Bendtsen F (2012) Infliximab and complications after colectomy in patients with ulcerative colitis. J Crohns Colitis 6(3):281–286
16. Selvasekar CR, Cima RR, Larson DW et al (2007) Effect of infliximab on short-term complications in patients undergoing operation for chronic ulcerative colitis. J Am Coll Surg 204(5):956–962; discussion 962–963

17. Mor IJ, Vogel JD, da Luz Moreira A et al (2008) Infliximab in ulcerative colitis is associated with an increased risk of postoperative complications after restorative proctocolectomy. Dis Colon Rectum 51(8):1202–1207
18. Gu J, Remzi FH, Shen B et al (2013) Operative strategy modifies risk of pouch-related outcomes in patients with ulcerative colitis on preoperative anti-tumor necrosis factor-α therapy. Dis Colon Rectum 56(11):1243–1252
19. Selvaggi F, Pellino G, Canonico S, Sciaudone G (2015) Effect of preoperative biologic drugs on complications and function after restorative proctocolectomy with primary ileal pouch formation: systematic review and meta-analysis. Inflamm Bowel Dis 21(1):79–92
20. Lightner AL, McKenna NP, Moncrief S et al (2017) Surgical outcomes in vedolizumab-treated patients with ulcerative colitis. Inflamm Bowel Dis 23(12):2197–2201

Surgical Treatment of Ulcerative Colitis: Indications and Techniques

9

9

Gilberto Poggioli, Lorenzo Gentilini, Maurizio Coscia, Luca Boschi, and Federica Ugolini

9.1 Introduction

With the exception of the sporadic use of an ileorectal anastomosis, until the early 1980s, the gold standard for surgery for patients with ulcerative colitis was a proctocolectomy with terminal ileostomy. In 1978, Parks and Nicholls introduced restorative proctocolectomy with ileal pouch-anal anastomosis (IPAA) for the first time [1]. This procedure is still considered the most common operation in patients with ulcerative colitis (UC) and is the gold standard procedure for the surgical management of this condition. Restorative proctocolectomy with ileal pouch-anal anastomosis removes the diseased large bowel preserving the natural manner of evacuation, eliminating the need for a permanent stoma, and providing good functional outcome and quality of life.

Although medical therapy has advanced in recent decades, evidence to date would suggest that there has been little change in the need for surgery [2]. In most of epidemiological studies, the cumulative risk for colectomy has ranged from 25% to 30% [3], with higher rates in patients having extensive and severe diseases [4]. A population-based study from Denmark has reported a colectomy rate of up to 60% at 10 years after diagnosis without significant changes in the surgical rate in the last 5 decades [5].

The surgical option should be evaluated by gastroenterologists, colorectal surgeons and patients. There is clear evidence that surgery provides good long-term disease control in many patients [2]. Surgery should be considered as an additional therapeutic alternative for patients with UC and not as a 'failure of

L. Gentilini (✉)
General Surgery Unit, Department of Digestive Diseases, S. Orsola-Malpighi Hospital
Bologna, Italy
e-mail: lorenzo.gentilini@aosp.bo.it

medical therapy'; this attitude could lead to optimal outcomes over the patient's lifetime; it is known that delay in operating may result in more advanced disease and hence more postoperative complications [2].

The main surgical indications for patients with UC can be classified into three groups: acute colitis with severe complications or not responding to medical therapy, chronic continuous disease causing steroid dependency in adults or impaired growth and/or delayed puberty in children and adolescents, and concomitant dysplasia and/or cancer of the colon.

9.2   Surgical Indications

9.2.1   Acute Colitis

All cases of acute colitis require close collaboration between the gastroenterologist and the colorectal surgeon. Absolute indications for surgery in cases of acute conditions are uncontrolled bleeding, perforation and toxic megacolon. The clinical presentation of UC has changed over time due to evolution in medical therapy. The success of conservative treatment causes a decrease in acute life-threatening complications, such as uncontrolled bleeding and toxic megacolon; therefore, acute colitis not responding to conservative treatment has increased [6]. Nowadays, acute colitis not responding to immunosuppressive therapy is the most frequent indication for non-elective surgery. There is clear evidence that a delay in appropriate surgery is detrimental to patient outcomes.

A staged procedure, initially with subtotal colectomy, is recommended in acute colitis in patients treated with high doses of steroids or undergoing rescue therapies with immunosuppressants or biologics [7].

Subtotal colectomy is a relatively safe procedure, even in critically ill patients. With subtotal colectomy, the diseased colon is removed while the rectal stump is left *in situ* to be removed subsequently. The handling of the rectal stump is still controversial. Leaving as little rectum as possible is not recommended because this approach imposes difficulties at subsequent proctectomy, with a probable increase in the risk of pelvic nerve injury. A first option is to divide the rectum at the level of the promontory and leave it closed in the pelvis; in this case, transanal drainage should be placed to prevent blowout due to retention. In order to avoid a possible leak of the rectal stump, with subsequent pelvic abscess or peritonitis, an alternative procedure is to bring the rectosigmoid up through the abdominal fascia (closed in the subcutaneous fat or as a mucous fistula). A mucous fistula results in an extra stoma for the patient, which may not be easily managed. For this reason, a closed rectal stump within the subcutaneous fat is preferred, although the skin should be allowed to heal through secondary intention in order to avoid wound infection or abscess formation in case of leaking of the suture. The latter option is considered very safe as no closed bowel is left within the abdomen.

Colectomy with an ileostomy allows the patients to recover from the colitis, with a quick return to health and nutritional status, and allows tapering of steroids. A preliminary subtotal colectomy also allows clarification of the pathology, definitively excluding Crohn's disease in order to plan subsequent surgery.

9.2.2   Chronic Colitis

Chronic continuous colitis is characterized by active disease despite maintenance therapy and often patients reported a steroid dependency. This condition frequently leads to the onset of steroid side effects with impairment of quality of life. Moreover, in young patients, a chronic inflammation could impair growth and/or delay puberty.

Even if patients with chronic disease are usually in better general condition than patients with acute colitis, they have often been under steroid or immuno-suppressant therapy for a long period of time. Prolonged medical therapy with high dose drugs (such as steroids, immunosuppressants, or biologics) significantly increases the risk of postoperative septic complications or anastomotic leaks [8–10].

According to these data, a staged procedure is also suggested for these patients. Patients with chronic colitis could be treated with both subtotal colectomy with terminal ileostomy and reconstruction at a later stage or with restorative proctocolectomy with ileoanal pouch and diverting ileostomy.

9.2.3   Dysplasia and Cancer

Dysplasia is associated with a high risk of neoplastic degeneration. The management of dysplasia in UC is based on a macroscopic pattern and microscopic characteristics of the lesion. Lesions could be macroscopically divided into polypoid, non-polypoid or macroscopically invisible while microscopic dysplasia is classified as indefinite, low grade or high grade. A polypoid lesion refers to a pedunculated or sessile lesion ≥2.5 mm which protrudes from the mucosa into the lumen. Polypoid dysplasia can be adequately treated by polypectomy provided the lesion can be completely excised, and there is no evidence of non-polypoid or invisible dysplasia elsewhere in the colon [6]. A non-polypoid lesion refers to lesions superficially elevated <2.5 mm, flat or depressed, velvety patches, plaques, irregular bumps and nodules, stricturing lesions, and broad-based masses, and may not be amenable to removal by colonoscopic polypectomy. Non-polypoid dysplastic lesions can be treated endoscopically only in selected cases. If complete resection can be achieved, with no evidence of non-polypoid or invisible dysplasia elsewhere in the colon, continued surveillance colonoscopy is reasonable. Every other patient with non-polypoid dysplasia should undergo surgery, regardless of the grade of dysplasia detected on bioptic analysis [6].

Macroscopically invisible dysplasia is considered to be a dysplasia identified from random biopsies. All patients with macroscopically invisible dysplasia should be referred to an endoscopist with expertise in inflammatory bowel disease (IBD) surveillance to determine whether a well-circumscribed lesion exists and can be resected, and to check for synchronous dysplasia. If a visible lesion is found in the same region of the colon as the invisible dysplasia, patients should be managed appropriately according to the polypoid or non-polypoid type of dysplasia identified. If no visible lesion is identified, and macroscopically invisible dysplasia is confirmed, its management depends on the grade of the initial dysplasia. High grade dysplasia is sufficient to warrant recommendation for colectomy. The management of low grade dysplasia is still controversial [6].

Recent data have reported an annual incidence in advanced cancer of 1.8% in patients with UC and low-grade dysplasia undergoing endoscopic surveillance. Moreover, in 12 surgical cohort studies, of the 450 patients who underwent colectomy for ulcerative colitis with low-grade dysplasia, 34 patients had synchronous colorectal cancer (17%). According to these findings, surgical treatment should also be suggested in cases of low-grade dysplasia [11].

A diagnosis of cancer of the colon or rectum in a patient with UC is an absolute indication for surgery. In cases of neoplastic degeneration, the patient should undergo proctocolectomy with, usually, an ileal pouch-anal anastomosis with or without diverting ileostomy. The proctocolectomy should be performed following oncological principles, such as the no-touch technique, high vascular ligation close to the origin of the vessels with lymphadenectomy. Proctectomy for cancer should be performed behind and laterally to the mesorectum in order to ensure total mesorectal excision (TME); this procedure is associated with a higher risk of pelvic nerve damage as compared to proctectomy inside the mesorectum (close mesorectal dissection), usually used for proctectomy in IBD patients. Proctectomy with TME is associated with better oncologic outcomes; however, patients undergoing TME report a higher incidence of 30-day postoperative complications and higher readmission rates. Moreover, patients undergoing a close mesorectal dissection report a better quality of life and higher results in functional scores [12].

The best type of ileoanal anastomosis in patients with neoplasia is still under debate. A hand-sewn anastomosis to the dentate line should be performed with mucosectomy of the rectal mucosa. This procedure is technically difficult and might damage the anal transitional zone, which is important for anal function, and does not guarantee the complete removal of the rectal mucosa. A double-stapled anastomosis is easier and faster, and it is associated with better long term functional outcomes [13, 14]. However, this type of anastomosis often leaves a rectal cuff with inflammation. The remaining rectal cuff should, however, be no more than 1–2 cm above the dentate line in order to minimize the mucosal surface at risk of malignant transformation.

A review of the literature reported the onset of cancer in the anal transitional zone, in patients undergoing both hand-sewn and stapled anastomosis [15]. For this reason, it could be concluded that mucosectomy does not rule out later development of cancer in the anorectal mucosa. Moreover, dysplasia or early cancer arising from the residual rectal mucosa after mucosectomy may not be easily noticeable and accessible because they develop between the pouch and the muscle layers of the cuff. Therefore, a stapled anastomosis is preferred and should be performed at the anorectal junction to avoid leaving behind diseased rectal mucosa which is prone to neoplastic changes.

In patients with advanced neoplasia of the colon with rectum sparing, a staged procedure is suggested. A subtotal colectomy with terminal ileostomy is preferred for all patients who have to undergo chemotherapy after surgery. A restorative proctectomy with IPAA should be proposed at the end of adjuvant therapy.

9.3   Surgical Techniques

9.3.1   Restorative Proctocolectomy with IPAA

A restorative proctocolectomy with IPAA consists of removal of the entire colon, the dissection and removal of the rectum, the creation of an ileal pouch, and the anastomosis of the ileal pouch to the anal canal using a hand-sewn or stapled technique.

This operation can be performed in a single surgical procedure or in staged procedures. Various approaches have been described in the literature (see Chapter 8, Fig. 8.1).

In the single-stage procedure, the patient undergoes proctocolectomy with restorative ileal pouch-anal anastomosis without diverting ileostomy. With a two-stage procedure, the patient is first treated with a restorative proctocolectomy with a covering ileostomy and with subsequent ileostomy closure. In a two-stage modified procedure, the first surgical procedure is total abdominal colectomy, preserving the rectum; the second operation includes proctectomy and fashioning of the ileal pouch-anal anastomosis without diverting ileostomy. In a three-stage procedure, the patient initially undergoes total abdominal colectomy, subsequent proctectomy with IPAA and covering ileostomy and, finally, an ileostomy closure is performed.

The best surgical approach should be evaluated on the basis of the patient's clinical condition, surgical indication (elective or urgent surgery) and preoperative medical therapy. Patients with chronic remittent colitis or long-standing disease with a diagnosis of concomitant dysplasia or cancer, undergoing elective surgery, without major medical therapy could undergo a single- or a two-stage procedure. Patients with compromised clinical status, undergoing urgent surgery or treated with high dose steroids or biologics prior to surgery could benefit from a first surgical procedure of total abdominal colectomy; the restoration of intestinal continuity should be postponed to a second procedure. For these patients, a 2-stage modified or a 3-stage procedure should be suggested.

9.3.2   Proctocolectomy

A total proctocolectomy is necessary for complete removal of the diseased colon. The first stage of the operation is abdominal colectomy. Abdominal colectomy is a simple and safe procedure. The entire colon must be mobilized from its retroperitoneal attachments, and a peripheral section of vascular pedicles should be constructed (only in the presence of *coexistent colon cancer*, should adherence to traditional standards of oncological resection be maintained). The ileocolic vessels must be preserved to ensure good vascularization of the ileal pouch; moreover, the presence of ileocolic vessels is necessary for the lengthening of the ileum required in the case of a hand-sewn anastomosis. The ileum must be transected immediately proximal to the ileocecal valve.

In a 2-stage modified or a 3-stage procedure, total abdominal colectomy should be performed, dividing the colon at the sigmoid rectal junction. The remaining rectum can be managed in different ways. In Hartmann's Pouch procedure, the rectum is divided at the level of the promontory and left closed in the pelvis. In this case, the rectum should be drained with a transanal drainage in order to prevent blowout due to retention. Hartmann's pouch procedure is associated with greater difficulty in the subsequent proctectomy, having higher rates of postoperative complications and pelvic autonomic nerve injuries. In order to reduce postoperative complications and nerve injuries in the subsequent proctectomy, the rectal stump could be divided at the rectosigmoid junction and fixed to the abdominal wall. The rectal stump could be fixed open as a mucous fistula or it could be closed.

With the proctectomy, the rectum should be completely removed and transected at the top of the anal columns, preserving the anal sensory epithelium leaving a 1–2 cm anal transitional zone. During the proctectomy, it is important to avoid injury to the pelvic autonomic nerves; the majority of patients are young and the preservation of sexual function is clearly mandatory. The proctectomy could be performed with either a close rectal dissection or mesorectal excision [1, 16].

In the presence of or when there is suspicion of dysplasia or cancer, a complete total mesorectal excision (TME) is recommended. Under benign conditions, a close rectal dissection could be adopted. This last approach reduces the risk of pelvic nerve damage and ensures better long-term functional outcome [12]; however, a dissection in this plane is less straightforward as it is not the bloodless plane encountered during a mesorectal dissection. A close mesorectal dissection of the upper rectum may protect the hypogastric nerves and reduce the incidence of retrograde ejaculation [17]. It is crucial not to violate the presacral fascia posteriorly where the lateral and presacral veins can be damaged. Nerve injury leading to impotence is sustained during the anterolateral dissection of the rectum; dissection of this region is similar in both techniques [18].

Anteriorly and laterally, the dissection should stay close to the rectum to avoid any nerve injury.

An anterior dissection is carried out at the lower border of the prostate gland or lower one-third of the vagina. Direct visualization of the seminal vesicles and most of the vagina should be possible.

Denonvilliers' fascia is preserved in patients without a carcinoma. Mobilization is continued until the coccyx is palpable posteriorly and complete circumferential mobilization of the rectum is obtained to the level of the elevators. A transanal digital evaluation with the tip of a finger is done to mark the level of rectal transaction.

9.3.3   Creation of an Ileal Pouch

The terminal ileus must be used for fashioning an ileal reservoir. The initial report of IPAA described a hand-sewn pouch with an "S" configuration [1]. The S is created using 3 limbs of 12 to 15 cm of terminal small bowel with a 2–3 cm exit conduit (about 50 cm of ileum all together). The ileum segments are approximated by continuous seromuscular sutures. An enterotomy is performed in an S shape. Continuous running full thickness sutures are applied to the two posterior anastomotic lines. Subsequently, the anterior wall is closed using continuous seromuscular sutures. Finally, it can be reinforced using interrupted sutures (Fig. 9.1).

The S pouch was initially described with an efferent limb of 3 cm [1]. Many patients treated with this procedure have reported evacuation problems, leading to the need for pouch intubation in up to 50% of cases [19]. Due to evacuation obstruction, the efferent limb of the S pouch has subsequently been shortened to try to reduce the incidence of this complication.

Surgical evolution and the introduction of the use of stapling techniques have led to a multitude of options for constructing pouches. These include the J, W, K, H, B, and U pouch [19–24].

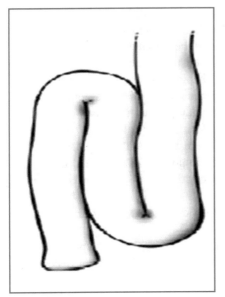

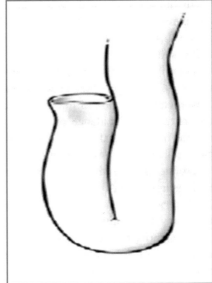

Fig. 9.1 S pouch   Fig. 9.2 J-pouch

Utsunomiya introduced the J-pouch. The J-pouch is constructed from the terminal 30–40 cm of small intestine. This ileum segment is folded into two 15- or 20-cm segments which must be sutured together side to side. This suture can be executed using two 2 cartridges of an ILA 100 linear stapler introduced at the pouch apex by an enterotomy; alternatively, this can be also hand-sewn. Finally, the blind loop of the J-pouch must be closed using a linear stapler and is usually then reinforced. A check of the staple lines for hemostasis is recommended.
Originally proposed to be 15 cm in length, pouches have subsequently been increased up to 20 cm. However, larger dimensions have been associated with pouch retention and difficulties in emptying. In effect, a J-pouch should range between 15–18 cm and be tailored to patient size. (Fig. 9.2).

The W-pouch was proposed by Nicholls and Pezim in 1985 [19], its potential advantages being a lower frequency of defecation and no requirement for pouch intubation. This design joins the advantages of both the J- and the S-pouches; however, it is technically more difficult to construct and more time-consuming. Moreover, its bulkiness may also result in greater difficulty in placing the pouch into a narrow pelvis. Similarly, to the S-pouch, the W-pouch must also be hand-sewn using approximately 50 cm of terminal ileum (Fig. 9. 3).

The remaining pouch designs were not completely validated by subsequent studies and did not reach wide diffusion in clinical practice.

Data from the literature have reported similar results between J-, S- and W-pouches. A meta-analysis [25] including 18 studies with 1519 patients undergoing restorative proctocolectomy with J-, S- or W-pouches analyzed the

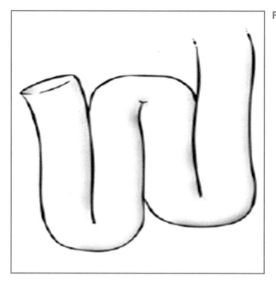

Fig. 9.3 W-pouch

differences in term of postoperative complications and functional outcomes between the three different pouch designs. No significant differences have been reported in postoperative complications including leak, stricture, pelvic sepsis, pouchitis, small bowel obstruction and pouch failure. According to functional outcomes, patients with a J-pouch reported more bowel movements than those treated with either the S- or the W-pouch. However, patients with S- or W-pouches reported more difficulty in pouch evacuation and frequently required the use of enemas or intubation. Seepage and incontinence were similar among the three types of pouch design.

Four randomized controlled trials have been published comparing J- and W-pouches. Two trials, one of 60 and one of 33 patients, have shown no differences in function between J- and W-pouches at up to 12 months of follow-up [26, 27]. Two additional trials of 24 and 50 patients each showed a mean daily defecation frequency higher in patients treated with a J-pouch which was associated with an increased use of antimotility drugs [28, 29].

It can be concluded that pouch function is not influenced by pouch design while it is very important to avoid injury to the anal sphincter so as to ensure pouch compliance and to maintain anal reflex. No superiority has been identified between pouch design; however, the J-pouch is technically easier to create and results in good function without the need for pouch intubation, and it is actually the most used in the world (more than 95% of surgeons use this pouch design). The S-pouch and W-pouch require hand-sewing; hence, they are more time consuming. The S-pouch is actually preferred when a J-pouch will not reach into the pelvis without tension, and a lengthening of the ileum is not possible or not sufficient.

9.3.4 Lengthening of the Ileum

Successful pouch surgery is based on a tension-free anastomosis between the ileal pouch and the anus. To reduce anastomotic tension, the small bowel mesentery should be mobilized adequately as far as the third part of the duodenum and all adhesions due to previous surgical procedures should be dissected [16]. The anastomotic tension can be estimated by grasping the apex of the pouch and simulating the tension produced by pulling it down to the level of the anastomosis. Moreover, a tension-free anastomosis can be obtained when the apex of the pouch reaches the inferior border of the pubic symphysis [16].

In some patients, it may be difficult to obtain enough length of the small intestine to allow a tension-free anastomosis with the anal canal. In cases of tension, a lengthening of the ileum must be performed to prevent anastomotic early or long-term complications, such as early anastomotic leaks or long-term anastomotic stenosis.

The lengthening of the ileum can be obtained in different ways. Division of either the terminal superior mesenteric artery (distal to the origin of the ileocolic vessel) or the ileocolic artery can be performed to additionally reduce tension and provide extra length, providing that the vascularity of the ileum is confirmed. Sufficient vasculature guaranteed by the residual vessel must be evaluated by clamping the vessels to be dissected before the division. Ileocolic division can provide an extra 3–7 cm of length. If it is not enough, the superior mesenteric artery can be divided distally to the origin of the ileocolic vessel. This procedure can be performed safely without impact on complication rates or functional outcomes if good vascularization is ensured by the ileocolic artery [30].

If there is still tension after these maneuvers, the peritoneal tissue between the vessel loop of the ileocolic and superior mesenteric artery can be excised using translumination by means of "mesenteric windows". Small anterior and posterior peritoneal incisions over the superior mesenteric vessels border can also be made as an additional maneuver.

Finally, the use of an S-pouch may result in an additional gain of 2 to 3 cm in length. The advantage of the S-pouch is an extra couple of centimeters in length as compared with other pouch configurations; this may be important when there are concerns regarding the ability to perform a tension-free IPAA [30].

9.3.5 Ileoanal Anastomosis

An ileoanal anastomosis can be performed using either a stapled or a hand-sewn technique. In their first report on restorative proctocolectomy, Parks and Nicholls proposed a hand-sewn anastomosis. The original procedure has changed over time, in particular, with the introduction of staplers.

A hand-sewn ileal pouch anal anastomosis must be performed with a muco-sectomy of the anal canal. With mucosectomy the entire anorectal mucosa must be removed from the dentate line up to the level of transaction of the rectum during proctectomy. A mucosectomy can be performed by placing an anal re-tractor and using submucosal injection of a solution of adrenalin (1:100,000) to raise the anorectal mucosa off the underlying muscle. In this way, it is possible to remove the diseased mucosa without damage to the anal sphincter (Fig. 9.4).

Subsequently, the anastomosis between the pouch and the anal canal must be performed at the dentate line with sutures placed radially, incorporating a small bit of internal anal sphincter and the apex of the J-pouch or the exit conduit of the S-pouch.

In cases of hand-sewn anastomosis, the pouch must be placed more distally in the pelvis when compared to stapled anastomosis. Therefore, good lengthening of the ileum must be obtained in all patients undergoing a hand-sewn procedure in order to ensure a tension-free anastomosis.

In the case of both hand-sewn and stapled anastomoses, great care must be taken to ensure that the surrounding tissues are not incorporated into the anastomosis, especially the posterior vaginal wall. In order to avoid the onset of pouch vaginal fistulas in patients undergoing hand-sewn anastomosis, anterior suturing should not be too deep in females. After removing the anal retractor, the sutures previously made can be tied. The anastomosis can be checked using colored saline introduced through the anus.

In most of cases of hand-sewn anastomoses, a diverting ileostomy is recommended. The ileostomy should be fashioned to the right lower quadrant of the abdomen; the site of the diverting ileostomy must be marked before the surgical procedure in order to identify the correct position of the stoma which would be comfortable for the patient. The loop ileostomy should pass through the rectus muscle of the abdominal wall to prevent incisional hernia.

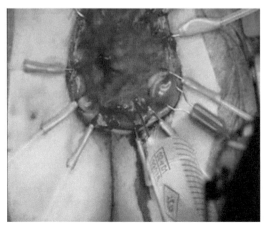

Fig. 9.4 Anal retractor and adrenaline injections

A stapled IPAA can be performed using either single- or double-stapled procedures.

In the single-stapled approach the anvil of the stapler could be placed at the apex of the pouch and secured with a purse string suture. A distal purse string must be applied to the anorectal stump and tightened on the surgical circular stapler inserted transanally. Finally, the anastomosis can be performed with the use of a circular stapler.

In the double-stapled technique, the distal anorectal stump is closed using a linear stapler, and the specimen is divided above the staple line. The anvil of the stapler is placed at the apex of the pouch and fixed with a purse string suture. The circular stapler must be inserted into the anus and moved into the anorectal stump up to the stapled line. The pin of the circular stapler must exit through the stapled line, and the two ends of the stapler can be approximated. Before firing with the stapler, the correct orientation of the small bowel must be checked to prevent twisting of the pouch on its mesentery. As for hand-sewn anastomosis, the integrity of the anastomosis should be checked. The double stapled procedure is easier and faster and actually is the most widely used. (Fig. 9.5).

In stapled anastomosis, the right distance from the dentate line is very important; the stapler must be placed at about 3 cm from dental line. In this way, a cuff of the anal transition zone is left in place with residual columnar mucosa. If the anastomosis is too low, it could damage the internal sphincter with subsequent incontinence. A long anorectal stump left in place leads to a diseased cuff which, in turn, could lead to the onset of cuffitis.

Ileostomy can be omitted only in selected patients, where the risk of the development of anastomotic complications is low.

In all patients with or without a diverting ileostomy transanal drainage is recommended. Its purpose is to avoid retention of fluids in the pouch which could create tension on the suture of the body of the reservoir or on the anastomosis. This drainage should be placed through the anus into the body of the pouch and fixed to the perineal skin; it should be left in place up to 4 to 5 days and irrigated with saline.

Prior to an ileostomy closure an endoscopy or a water-contrasted pouchogram is suggested to check the integrity of both the pouch and the anastomosis. If no complications are identified, closure of the ileostomy can be performed in 2 to 3 months after restorative proctocolectomy.

Randomized trials did not find any differences between stapled or hand-sewn anastomoses as regards early septic postoperative complications; both the procedures can be considered feasible and safe [31, 32]. No differences have been reported regarding onset of dysplasia or cancer in the anal transition zone between patients undergoing stapled or hand-sewn anastomoses [15].

Poorer functional outcomes have been described in patients treated with hand-sewn anastomosis. This could be due to a combination of mechanical trauma to the anal sphincter and removal of the anal transition zone. The anal

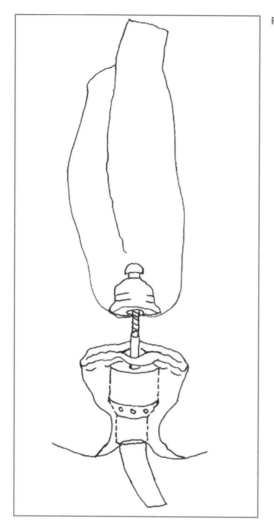

Fig. 9.5 Double-stapled anastomosis

sphincter could be damaged when using an anal retractor or during dissection for mucosectomy. Bowel movements during the day or at night are similar in patients treated with stapled or hand-sewn anastomoses. However, patients treated with the hand-sewn technique report higher urgency and incontinence (both seepage and soiling) than patients with a stapled anastomosis. Subsequently, the use of protective pads and the incidence of perianal irritation are more frequent in patients with a hand-sewn anastomosis. Higher anal-canal resting pressure and squeeze pressure are also found when the stapled technique was used [31, 32]. According to these data, a hand-sewn anastomosis is associated with more social restrictions, and patients report lower scores regarding quality of life [13, 14].

Currently, stapler IPAA is the preferred technique because it is easier and quicker to perform and is associated with better long-term functional outcomes. A hand-sewn anastomosis is preferred in patients with a failure of the stapled technique or in patients requiring redo surgery.

9.3.6   Diverting Ileostomy

Septic postoperative early complications are difficult to treat in patients undergoing restorative proctocolectomy and should be avoided. Anastomotic leaks or pelvic abscess can lead to poor long-term functional outcomes. In these patients, bowel movements do not change significantly while incontinence rates, need for protective pads and medication usage are increased to a greater extent than in patients without postoperative complications. Similarly, lifestyle restrictions also occur more frequently [33]. Moreover, patients with postoperative septic complications have a higher risk of pouch failure (permanent diversion or pouch excision) [33]. The role of defunctioning ileostomy for the prevention of postoperative complications is still under debate.

Various studies have concluded that a diverting ileostomy does not reduce the incidence of postoperative septic complications, such as anastomotic or suture line leaks; however, the presence of a diverting ileostomy is helpful in managing the septic complications [34]. An anastomotic leak after restorative proctocolectomy with a loop ileostomy is frequently subclinical or associated with reduced clinical impact, and it could heal without additional surgery. Conversely, randomized control trials comparing patients with or without diverting ileostomy have reported a lower incidence of septic complications and anastomotic leaks in patients with a diverting ileostomy [34]. However, the fashioning of a diverting ileostomy can be associated with postoperative clinical advantages, although it could also lead to postoperative complications.

The formation of an ileostomy is associated with its own set of potential complications, both mechanical and functional. Of the mechanical complications, stoma retraction, stoma prolapse, fistula formation with abdominal abscess or abscess of the abdominal wall or bowel obstruction related to the stoma have been described. In patients with a diverting ileostomy, functional complications – such as peristomal irritation, incomplete diversion of high intestinal output with subsequent dehydration or kidney failure – could occur.

Moreover, it should also be considered that stoma reversal is another abdominal procedure for the patient and this procedure can be associated with postoperative complications. In a study conducted on more than 1500 patients undergoing ileostomy reversal after IPAA, small-bowel obstruction (6.4%), wound infection (1.5%), abdominal septic complications (1%) and enterocutaneous fistulas (0.6%) has been described [35]. According to these considerations, the decision regarding fashioning a diverting ileostomy must balance the complications of ileostomy construction and closure against the risk and complications of pelvic sepsis.

A diverting ileostomy can be omitted only in selected cases, such as in patients who are in good health, not on chronic steroid or immunosuppressant therapy and having an absolutely tension-free stapled anastomosis. Ileostomy closure can be performed two or three months after restorative proctocolectomy, after a satisfactory water-soluble contrast pouch study or endoscopy.

References

1. Parks AG, Nicholls RJ (1978) Proctocolectomy without ileostomy for ulcerative colitis. Br Med J 2(6130):85–88
2. Mowat C, Cole A, Windsor A et al; IBD Section of the British Society of Gastroenterology (2011) Guidelines for the management of inflammatory bowel disease in adults. Gut 60(5):571–607
3. Henriksen M, Jahnsen J, Lygren I et al; IBSEN Study Group (2006) Ulcerative colitis and clinical course: results of a 5-year population-based follow-up study (the IBSEN study). Inflamm Bowel Dis 12(7):543–550
4. Cottone M, Scimeca D, Mocciaro F et al (2008) Clinical course of ulcerative colitis. Dig Liver Dis 40(Suppl 2):S247–S252
5. Jess T, Riis L, Vind I et al (2007) Changes in clinical characteristics, course, and prognosis of inflammatory bowel disease during the last 5 decades: a population-based study from Copenhagen, Denmark. Inflamm Bowel Dis 13(4):481–489
6. Teeuwen PH, Stommel MW, Bremers AJ et al (2009) Colectomy in patients with acute colitis: a systematic review. J Gastrointest Surg 13(4):676–686
7. Magro F, Gionchetti P, Eliakim R et al; European Crohn's and Colitis Organisation [ECCO] (2017) Third European evidence-based consensus on diagnosis and management of ulcerative colitis. Part 1: definitions, diagnosis, extra-intestinal manifestations, pregnancy, cancer surveillance, surgery, and ileo-anal pouch disorders. J Crohns Colitis 11(6):649–670
8. Ehteshami-Afshar S, Nikfar S, Rezaie A, Abdollahi M (2011) A systematic review and meta-analysis of the effects of infliximab on the rate of colectomy and post-operative complications in patients with inflammatory bowel disease. Arch Med Sci 7(6):1000–1012
9. Selvasekar CR, Cima RR, Larson DW et al (2007) Effect of infliximab on short-term complications in patients undergoing operation for chronic ulcerative colitis. J Am Coll Surg 204(5):956–962
10. Mor IJ, Vogel JD, da Luz Moreira A et al (2008) Infliximab in ulcerative colitis is associated with an increased risk of postoperative complications after restorative proctocolectomy. Dis Colon Rectum 51(8):1202–1207
11. Fumery M, Dulai PS, Gupta S et al (2017) Incidence, risk factors, and outcomes of colorectal cancer in patients with ulcerative colitis with low-grade dysplasia: a systematic review and meta-analysis. Clin Gastroenterol Hepatol 15(5):665–674
12. Bartels SA, Gardenbroek TJ, Aarts M et al (2015) Short-term morbidity and quality of life from a randomized clinical trial of close rectal dissection and total mesorectal excision in ileal pouch-anal anastomosis. Br J Surg 102(3):281–287
13. Gozzetti G, Poggioli G, Marchetti F et al (1994) Functional outcome in handsewn versus stapled ileal pouch-anal anastomosis. Am J Surg 168(4):325–329
14. Kirat HT, Remzi FH, Kiran RP, Fazio VW (2009) Comparison of outcomes after handsewn versus stapled ileal pouch-anal anastomosis in 3,109 patients. Surgery 146(4):723–729; discussion 729–730

15. Um JW, M'Koma AE (2011) Pouch-related dysplasia and adenocarcinoma following restorative proctocolectomy for ulcerative colitis. Tech Coloproctol 15(1):7–16
16. Ballantyne GH, Pemberton JH, Beart RW Jr et al (1985) Ileal J pouch-anal anastomosis. Current technique. Dis Colon Rectum 28(3):197–202
17. Nicholls RJ, Lubowski DZ (1987) Restorative proctocolectomy: the four loop (W) reservoir. Br J Surg 74(7):564–566
18. Lindsey I, George BD, Kettlewell GW, Mortensen NJ (2001) Impotence after mesorectal and close dissection for inflammatory bowel disease. Dis Colon Rectum 44(6):831–835
19. Nicholls RJ, Pezim ME (1985) Restorative proctocolectomy with ileal reservoir for ulcerative colitis and familial adenomatous polyposis: a comparison of three reservoir designs. Br J Surg 72(6):470–474
20. Utsunomiya J, Iwama T, Imajo M et al (1980) Total colectomy, mucosal proctectomy, and ileoanal anastomosis. Dis Colon Rectum 23(7):459–466
21. Hallgren T, Fasth S, Nordgren S et al (1989) Manovolumetric characteristics and functional results in three different pelvic pouch designs. Int J Colorectal Dis 4(3):156–160
22. Fonkalsrud EW (1987) Update on clinical experience with different surgical techniques of the endorectal pull-through operation for colitis and polyposis. Surg Gynecol Obstet 165(4):309–316
23. Slors JF, Taat CW, Brummelkamp WH (1989) Ileal pouch-anal anastomosis without rectal muscular cuff. Int J Colorectal Dis 4(3):178–181
24. Nelson RL, Prasad ML, Pearl RK, Abcarian H (1991) Inverted U-pouch construction for restoration of function in patients with failed straight ileoanal pull-throughs. Dis Colon Rectum 34(11):1040–1042
25. Lovegrove RE, Heriot AG, Constantinides V et al (2007) Meta-analysis of short-term and long-term outcomes of J, W and S ileal reservoirs for restorative proctocolectomy. Colorectal Dis 9(4):310–320
26. Johnston D, Williamson ME, Lewis WG et al (1996) Prospective controlled trial of duplicated (J) versus quadruplicated (W) pelvic ileal reservoirs in restorative proctocolectomy for ulcerative colitis. Gut 39(2):242–247
27. Keighley MR, Yoshioka K, Kmiot W (1988) Prospective randomized trial to compare the stapled double lumen pouch and the sutured quadruple pouch for restorative proctocolectomy. Br J Surg 75(10):1008–1011
28. Selvaggi SF, Giuliani A, Gallo C et al (2000) Randomized, controlled trial to compare the J-pouch and W-pouch configurations for ulcerative colitis in the maturation period. Dis Colon Rectum 43(5):615–620
29. Lumley J, Stevenson A, Stitz R (2002) Prospective randomized study of J vs. W pouches in ulcerative colitis. Dis Colon Rectum 45:A5
30. Smith L, Friend WG, Medwell SJ (1984) The superior mesenteric artery. The critical factor in the pouch pull-through procedure. Dis Colon Rectum 27(11):741–744
31. Reilly WT, Pemberton JH, Wolff BG et al (1997) Randomized prospective trial comparing ileal pouch-anal anastomosis by excising the anal mucosa to ileal pouch-anal anastomosis performed by preserving the anal mucosa. Ann Surg 225(6):666–676; discussion 676–677
32. Hallgren TA, Fasth SB, Øresland TO, Hultén LA (1995) Ileal pouch anal function after endoanal mucosectomy and handsewn ileoanal anastomosis compared with stapled anastomosis without mucosectomy. Eur J Surg 161(12):915–921
33. Farouk R, Dozois RR, Pemberton JH, Larson D (1998) Incidence and subsequent impact of pelvic abscess after ileal pouch-anal anastomosis for chronic ulcerative colitis. Dis Colon Rectum 41(10):1239–1243
34. Hüser N, Michalski CW, Erkan M et al (2008) Systematic review and meta-analysis of the role of defunctioning stoma in low rectal cancer surgery. Ann Surg 248(1):52–60
35. Wong KS, Remzi FH, Gorgun E et al (2005) Loop ileostomy closure after restorative proctocolectomy: outcome in 1,504 patients. Dis Colon Rectum 48(2):243–250

Surgical Treatment of Ulcerative Colitis: Laparoscopy and New Minimally Invasive Techniques

10

Gilberto Poggioli and Matteo Rottoli

10.1 Introduction

Over the last two decades, the benefits of the minimally invasive approach in treating colorectal cancer have been widely demonstrated. Only a few large randomized clinical trials and subsequent reviews have shown the indisputable short-term advantages when resection was performed laparoscopically [1–3]. Shorter hospital stay, less postoperative pain, less blood loss and faster return to an oral diet are only a few of the variables which are significantly improved after a laparoscopic procedure. The long-term advantages, such as a lower incidence of incisional hernia and adhesional bowel obstruction, as well as better cosmesis, are also observed.

These benefits are important especially in the population of ulcerative colitis (UC) patients who are usually young and likely to undergo more than one surgical procedure during their lifetime. In fact, despite improvements in the conservative management of ulcerative colitis, surgery is still required in up to 40% of patients [4, 5]. Improved medical therapy has led to a decrease in emergency colectomy (either from uncontrolled bleeding or toxic megacolon) from 70% to 10% of patients, thereby increasing the opportunity for performing an elective laparoscopic procedure.

Obviously, the indications for a 1-, 2- or 3-stage restorative proctocolectomy with ileal pouch-anal anastomosis (IPAA) are the same, regardless of the surgical access. However, theoretically, the minimally invasive approach, which is associated with a faster recovery and a lower incidence of postoperative

M. Rottoli (✉)
Department of Medical and Surgical Sciences, University of Bologna, S. Orsola-Malpighi Hospital
Bologna, Italy
e-mail: matteo.rottoli2@unibo.it

G. Poggioli (Ed), *Ulcerative Colitis*,
Updates in Surgery
DOI: 10.1007/978-88-470-3977-3_10, © Springer-Verlag Italia 2019

complications, is ideal not only for a fit, young patient undergoing an elective procedure, but also, and especially, in the case of an ill and fragile patient.

A Cochrane review published in 2009 showed that laparoscopic IPAAs were associated with increased operative time and costs, and better cosmesis [6]. A subsequent review by the American College of Surgeons National Surgical Quality Improvement Program (NSQIP) analyzed the outcomes of 676 IPAA procedures, 50% of which were performed laparoscopically. The analysis showed that the laparoscopic approach was associated with a lower rate of major (odds ratio [OR] 0.67, p 0.04) and minor (OR 0.44, p 0.01) postoperative complications while the hospital stay was similar between the procedures [7].

Moreover, two recent studies have shown significantly improved female fecundity after minimally invasive IPAA [8, 9]. Based on the evidence, the European Crohn's and Colitis Organisation (ECCO) have recently released a statement in their latest guidelines highlighting the safety, feasibility and advantages of laparoscopy in the treatment of UC [10].

However, in order to be effective and minimize the operative time and the rate of intra- and postoperative complications, minimally invasive surgery requires an unavoidable learning curve. Over ten years ago, a report from the Cleveland Clinic Foundation in Ohio showed that the expertise of the surgeon in the open procedure was strictly related to the onset of perioperative morbidity and long-term pouch failure [11]. The minimum number of pouch procedures necessary to obtain a significant reduction in pouch failure was calculated in 40 and 31 patients for stapled and hand-sewn IPAAs, respectively. More recently, the same team analyzed the outcomes in relationship to the learning curve during laparoscopic IPAA [12]. The authors showed that high volume surgeons were able to significantly decrease the operative time during total proctocolectomies and, more important, the rate of postoperative pelvic sepsis. The latter complication should be seen as the most important postoperative outcome as several reports have shown that sepsis is correlated with long-term poor functional outcomes and pouch failure [13].

The importance of continuous training in the laparoscopic approach and performing a large number of consecutive procedures is undisputable. High volume centers (and surgeons) are more likely to minimize the risk of morbidity and to optimize the outcomes of their patients while the surgeons who perform these procedures infrequently over a long period of time (regardless of the total number of operations) might not be able to improve the results of the surgery, either short or long term.

In this regard, it should be stressed that the first step towards the improvement of outcomes after IPAA is the centralization of these procedures since, currently, only a few national centers are able to provide surgical treatment for a large volume of patients.

10.2   Subtotal Colectomy

The indications for subtotal colectomy in ulcerative colitis are a refractory course of disease and urgent complications, such as bleeding, perforation and toxic megacolon. Ulcerative colitis complicated by neoplastic transformation usually suggests the need for a restorative proctocolectomy. However, in cases of frail patients, a colectomy would be the best choice in order to avoid any anastomosis.

Despite the fact that the feasibility and the advantages of the minimally invasive technique have been demonstrated [14], until recently more than half of colectomies were performed using an open approach (data from national databases in the USA, 2005–2010) [15, 16].

While the Cochrane review published in 2009 did not reveal any great benefit of laparoscopy in UC patients, except for a reduced hospital stay [6], more recent studies have confirmed faster recovery after laparoscopy and, more importantly, a reduced incidence of major and minor complications [7, 17]. Other authors have confirmed a significant decrease in surgical site infections after laparoscopic colectomies [18], as well as a drastic decline in the postoperative ileus rate [14]. A possible improvement in the onset of thromboembolic events was pointed out by studies comparing laparoscopic and open colectomies for UC [19], although such a difference was likely to be due to the different case-mix of patients undergoing the open or key-hole procedure.

The role of laparoscopy in the emergency treatment of UC (in particular, toxic megacolon and perforation) is still under debate. While technically feasible, the increased operative time, the risk of bowel perforation due to the fragility of the dilated bowel, and the difficulty of achieving a proper washout of the abdominal cavity in case of perforation, remain strong factors which suggest proceeding with an open subtotal colectomy. additional randomized studies might clarify the safety of the laparoscopic approach in this specific subset of patients.

10.2.1 Technique

The patient is placed in a lithotomy position. Specific devices (bean bags, shoulder supports, specific gripping mattresses) are used to provide safe support to the patient during the movement of the operating table. A 13–15 mmHg pneumoperitoneum is established after the open insertion of a 12-mm supraumbilical port. Another four 12-mm ports are positioned in a rhomboid shape in the epigastrium and the suprapubic, left and right flank areas. While 5-mm ports could be used, it has been found that 12-mm trocars are preferred as they allow the insertion of larger instruments (staplers and clip applicators) or swabs when needed, especially in the case of bleeding. Should a proctocolectomy be performed, moving the right flank port inferiorly towards the iliac spine is suggested in order for the surgeon to be more comfortable during the proctectomy. While the hand-assisted technique has been reported in the literature, it does not provide any real benefit due to the longer incision and poorer laparoscopic visualization. However, such an approach could improve the confidence of the operator, especially at the early stage of the learning curve.

The dissection can be started in a clockwise or anti-clockwise direction, depending on surgeon preference. Similarly, a lateral to medial or a medial to lateral approach to the mesentery division could be used. In cases of UC not complicated by cancer, part of the mesentery can be left in situ in order to minimize the risk of injury to the retroperitoneal structures or the risk of major bleeding, especially during dissection of the transverse mesocolon. Depending on the location of the dissection, a mixed approach was chosen. However, it might be preferable to start with lateral mobilization of the bowel in order to increase the extension of the mesentery and allow a safe dissection.

Following the steps of open colectomies, dissection can begin from the right colon and proceed in a clockwise direction. The right colon should first be mobilized laterally up to the splenic flexure, being careful not to damage the duodenum. At the level of the ileocecal valve, the mesentery should be dissected very close to the bowel in order to preserve the ileocolic vessels. Although a division of the ileocolic artery allows faster dissection [20], it should always be left intact (except, obviously, in the case of right colon cancer complicating the UC). In fact, while a standard, stapled J-pouch can easily be performed regardless of the ileocolic vascularization, should pouch revision surgery be needed in the future, mesentery lengthening could be necessary. In these cases, the superior mesenteric artery can be divided just distal to its ileocolic origin, allowing extension of the ileal mesentery by several centimeters which can be crucial, especially if a hand-sewn anastomosis is necessary.

Given the fact that these patients are usually young, and pouch complications requiring redo surgery might appear even after many years [21, 22], pre-emptive and cautious behavior must always be used. In some cases, in fact, the chance of a redo-pouch is frustrated by the absence of the alternative blood supply required to perform effective mesentery lengthening.

An alternative approach, preferred by many surgeons, is to first take down the splenic flexure in a lateral to medial fashion. This step has the advantage of prioritizing a potentially difficult passage, without requiring multiple moves of the surgeon. In this case, in fact, the operator stays on the right side of the patient, and after complete mobilization of the flexure, the dissection continues caudally to the level of the distal sigmoid colon. In the case of a subtotal colectomy, the inferior mesenteric artery should be preserved. This has two advantages: a better blood supply to the rectal stump (which might reduce the risk of ischemia or leak) and a faster identification of a "virgin" holy plane at the time of the proctectomy. Therefore, after the takedown of the lateral attachment of the left colon, the mesentery should be divided far from Toldt's fascia. The use of tissue-sealing devices utilizing advanced energy (either radiofrequency or ultrasound) allows safe hemostasis and faster dissection. In cases of a thick mesentery, a more cautious approach uses clips or plastic hem-o-locks for the vessels.

Management of the rectal stump has been under debate for decades [23–25]. Depending on surgeon preferences, the rectum could be either divided close to the rectosigmoid junction and abandoned in the abdomen, or more proximally at the level of the distal sigmoid colon and fixed to the abdominal wall in various ways. In particular, for the latter option, the rectosigmoid remnant can be left closed subcutaneously or open as a mucous fistula. No prospective comparative trials exist; a recent retrospective analysis showed that subcutaneous placement of the stump was associated with more frequent, although less severe, morbidity. In particular, the intraperitoneal closure was associated with leak and sepsis, requiring longer antibiotic treatment or a computed tomography-guided drainage [26].

Traditionally, either leaving the closed sigmoid remnant in the subcutaneous space or fashioning a mucous fistula is preferred. A transanal catheter is usually left in situ in order to drain the rectum and prevent blowout of the stump. Such a strategy could also be used to prevent the dehiscence of an intraperitoneal stump, as has been shown by other authors [27].

Once the left colon has been dealt with, the surgeon moves between the legs of the patient and proceeds with the transverse colon dissection. A reverse Trendelenburg position helps to obtain better exposure of the gastrocolic space.

The takedown of the omentum is optional and depends on surgeon preference. There is no evidence in the literature regarding the advantage of either of the approaches. The future use of the omentum as an omental flap in the case of a pouch-vaginal fistula, for example, can be a motive for preserving the omentum. Under some conditions (very thin or short omentum), it is just more practical to divide the gastroepiploic and gastrocolic ligaments and obtain proper mobilization of the transverse mesocolon. At this point, the mesocolon could be approached from the top, applying proper traction of the colon towards the right side of the patient, or from the bottom up. The former has the advantage of a safer division as the mesentery is stretched towards the operator and the application of the energy device (from the left flank port) is perpendicular to the mesentery and follows the line of dissection. On the other hand, the latter allows better visualization of the middle colic vessels and their branches, and approaching them more confidently. In any case, dividing the branches of the middle colic vessels distally is suggested in order to avoid any possible bleeding at the level of the inferior pancreatic edge, which could be very tricky to manage.

Depending on the fate of the rectal stump, the bowel can be divided either at the level of the terminal ileum (again, carefully avoiding the ileocolic vessels) and the specimen be extracted through a very small Pfannenstiel incision, or at the recto-sigmoid junction. In the latter case, the rectal stump is usually left in the abdomen, and the specimen can be removed through the same incision as the end ileostomy. The first technique is, however, preferred, as the longer recto-sigmoid stump is usually placed subcutaneously. The sigmoid can be divided outside the abdomen through the incision in order for it to be the proper length. As the mesentery is also taken down by the Alexis retractor, this approach has the advantage of more accurate hemostasis, in particular in the case of a bulky, inflamed mesocolon. End ileostomy is exteriorized through a pre-marked site in the right iliac fossa under laparoscopic vision. This should always be carried out as it is very easy for the terminal ileum to twist without the surgeon noticing it.

A large Foley catheter is subsequently positioned transanally in the rectal stump in order to facilitate drainage of fluids and decompression of the stump.

10.3 Restorative Proctectomy with Ileal Pouch-anal Anastomosis

10.3.1 Technique

Whether the proctocolectomy is performed during a one-stage procedure or following a previous subtotal colectomy, the trocar position and the technique are very similar to those of a low anterior resection for cancer (Fig. 10.1). The inferior mesenteric artery is mobilized from the posterior plane and can be divided distally. In the case of cancer or a high-grade dysplasia lesion in the left colon, an oncologic lymphadenectomy should be performed, and the vessels divided at the origin. A blunt dissection allows preservation of the posterior nerves, which should be carefully avoided in order to preserve the urinary and sexual function of the patient. The use of a latest generation laparoscope (in particular with 4K definition) greatly improves the identification of the small nerves visible on the sacral plane. The holy plane must be followed, first posteriorly and, subsequently, laterally and anteriorly. While, unlike in cancer patients, there is no risk of fibrosis secondary to neoadjuvant radiation, severe proctitis could sometimes mimic the same inflammation and make a clean dissection much more demanding.

Some surgeons claim that an intramesorectal dissection (close to the rectum) is safer in terms of nerve sparing and has the advantage of leaving some mesorectum on the presacral plane as a sort of cushion for the pouch. While there is no evidence that such an approach could provide any benefit for pouch function, a more difficult dissection, especially in the lower rectum, should be expected. Moreover, the risk of mesorectal bleeding and worse visualization of the pelvis discourage the use of this technique. A proper, nerve sparing total mesorectal excision (TME) allows the preservation of the sexual and urinary functions as long as the usual principles of mesorectal dissection are followed.

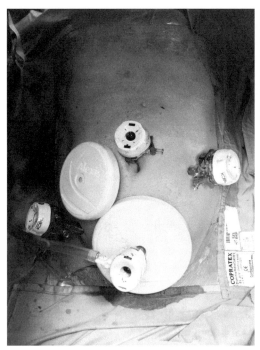

Fig. 10.1 Trocar position during laparoscopic restorative proctectomy and ileal pouch-anal anastomosis formation (small Alexis retractor is positioned after mobilization of the ileostomy; medium Alexis retractor is positioned after mobilization of the rectal stump, previously fixed to the abdominal wall)

It is advisable to maintain the dissection close to the rectum laterally and anteriorly in order not to damage the hypogastric nerves and to preserve the Denonvilliers' fascia (rectoprostatic fascia) in male patients.

Ulcerative colitis patients are more likely to have rectal prolapse, probably due to their bowel habits in the years before surgery. Proper rectal traction is therefore essential for providing a good exposure of the pelvic structure. A proper Trendelenburg position helps. However, the use of a 10-mm laparoscopic Babcock forceps inserted into the suprapubic port can be used to straighten the rectum cranially.

The dissection should be continued down to the level of the inferior rectal arteries, which are usually visible at the level of the levator ani plane. An endorectal digital examination will confirm the proper extension of the mesorectal excision. An excessive dissection through the pelvic floor should be avoided in order to preserve the vascularization of the rectal cuff and to avoid the division of the anorectum too close to the levators. On the other hand, it has been well recognized that laparoscopy is more likely to be associated with the tendency of leaving a long rectal stump, which would probably cause outlet obstruction of the pouch and require revision surgery in the future. This could be due to an insufficient dissection or to a difficult insertion of the laparoscopic stapler. In fact, despite the technological improvement of the staplers, a narrow pelvis and the limited articulation of the device is likely to force the surgeon to

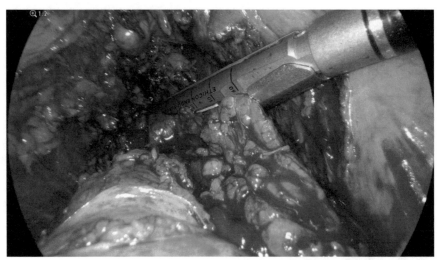

Fig. 10.2 A laparoscopic linear stapler is positioned at the level of the low rectum. The stapler line will be oblique, and multiple fires will be required

perform oblique and multiple staple lines (Fig. 10.2). This should be avoided, both for the possible consequence on pouch emptying and for the well-known increased risk of anastomotic leak [28].

As for other procedures, the first aim of the laparoscopic technique is to be at least non inferior in terms of outcomes to the open classic approach. Therefore, the same technique of rectal division performed in the last decades in our center (in over 1300 IPAA procedures) was adapted for the laparoscopic approach. The open, 30-mm linear stapler (DST series, TA Stapler, Medtronic, Minneapolis, MN, USA) has the unique advantage of a limited size, manual control of the retaining pin at the edge of the cartridge and, more importantly, the possibility of performing a perpendicular, singular staple line at the level of the low rectum.

The stapler could be inserted through a gel port or better in a cut glove finger which is mounted over a medium size Alexis port (Applied Medical, Rancho Santa Margarita, CA, USA), positioned in a small Pfannenstiel incision (Figs. 10.3–10.5). The glove reduces the risk of losing the pneumoperitoneum during the insertion and, at the same time, provides a wider range of movement of the stapler. The pneumoperitoneum is restored, and the stapler is positioned at the proper level of the rectum under laparoscopic vision (Fig. 10.6). This technique has been used several times during the latest laparoscopic IPAA anastomoses and has been found to be feasible, accurate and safe.

The only disadvantage of the TA stapler is the absence of cutting. However, this could easily be carried out using laparoscopic scissors or by placing the energy device just over the staple line.

The ileostomy is therefore divided, and the mesentery of the terminal ileum is mobilized cranially over the duodenum.

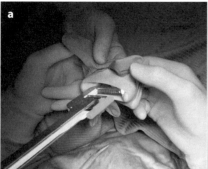
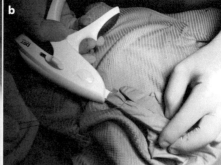
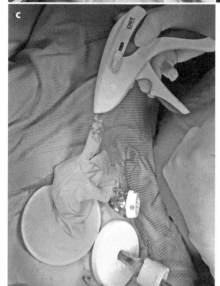

Fig. 10.3 A linear, open 30-mm stapler is inserted into a pre-cut glove, over the medium size Alexis retractor

The specimen and the terminal ileum (or the end ileostomy, once taken down) are extracted through the Alexis port (Fig. 10.7). A 15–20-cm J-pouch is constructed using two cartridges of a 100-mm linear stapler (ILA 100, Medtronic, Minneapolis, MN, USA) (Figs 10.8, 10.9). The internal line is checked for bleeding, and the anvil of the transanal circular stapler is inserted. Size-wise, the largest circular stapler allowed by the patient's anatomy is advised. A 31-mm stapler is usually found to be usable, and is likely to reduce the risk of IPAA stricture in the future (Fig. 10.10).

After the pneumoperitoneum is restored, the pouch is pulled down to the pelvis in order to confirm the absence of tension on the subsequent anastomosis. In case of any doubt, the mesentery of the terminal ileum is additionally mobilized. Should this not be enough, a proper mesentery lengthening procedure should be performed in order to ensure a tension-free anastomosis.

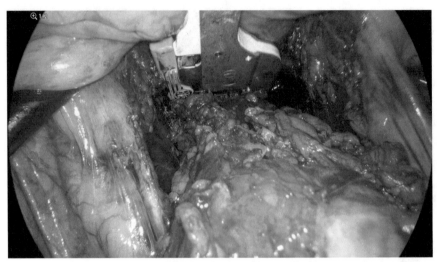

Fig. 10.4 The linear, 30-mm stapler is positioned at the right level of the low rectum. A single, perpendicular stapler line will be formed

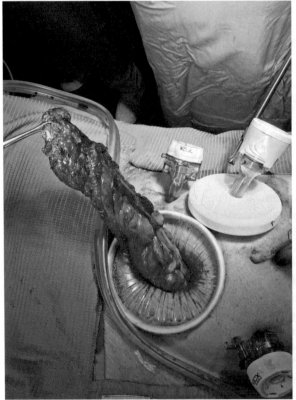

Fig. 10.5 After division, the rectum is removed through the suprapubic Alexis retractor

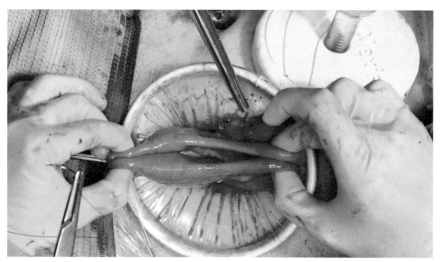

Fig. 10.6 Following laparoscopic mobilization, the terminal ileum is exteriorized through the retractor, and measured in order to create a J-pouch

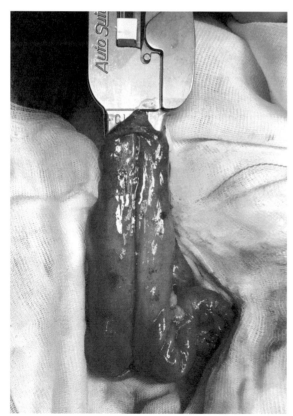

Fig. 10.7 The J-pouch is performed using two fires of an open, linear 100-mm stapler

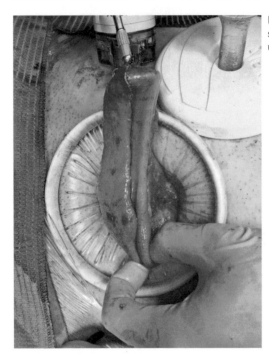

Fig. 10.8 The anvil of the circular stapler is positioned into the J-pouch using a purse-string suture

The pin of the transanal stapler is cautiously deployed and passes through the linear stapler line of the anal stump. It is important to avoid any excessive force on the line. Should the insertion of the stapler be tricky, 3 or 4 Foerster forceps could be placed on the quadrants at the level of the anocutaneous verge, providing effective and non-traumatic anal dilatation.

The IPAA is performed under vision and the orientation of the mesentery of the pouch is checked just before the stapler is closed. It is of utmost importance to follow the advancement of the pouch to the anal stump laparoscopically in order to avoid involvement of other pelvic structures in the sutures. In particular, in the case of female patients, particular attention should be paid to the vagina, as there is an elevated risk of causing an iatrogenic pouch-vaginal fistula. An air leak test is performed, the hemostasis is checked and a suction drain is left in the pelvis; a loop of proximal bowel is therefore exteriorized under laparoscopic vision as a diverting ileostomy. An ileostomy is routinely performed at the time of IPAA.

10.4   Future Developments

The outcomes of transanal TME for cancer have been evaluated in the past few years. Despite the different points of view and the required learning curve, recent reports show encouraging results regarding, in particular, conversion rate and intraoperative complications [29]. As a consequence of these preliminary good outcomes, the technique has been applied to restorative proctocolectomy [30, 31]. Hypothetically, the possible advantages of the various approaches are a better vision of the pelvis, especially in the lower part, and control of the level of the anastomosis.

A retrospective multicentric study has recently been published, comparing the outcomes of transanal versus transabdominal proctectomy with IPAA formation [32]. The study involved 97 patients undergoing the transanal approach, concluding that this technique was safe and was, in fact, associated with fewer complications as compared to the "standard" laparoscopic approach. Although these results open interesting scenarios for the future, caution is still necessary. The limits of the study, in fact, include the use of several different techniques (robotic, single-port, hand-assisted) from three centers as well as the decision to perform a close rectal dissection in a proportion of transanal-IPAA patients. Proper randomized clinical trials are required to confirm these initial findings.

Robotic surgery has also been investigated in the field of pouch surgery. There is limited evidence regarding the technique as applied to inflammatory bowel diseases [33–35]. A recent report from the Cleveland Clinic in Ohio showed good outcomes after robotic restorative proctectomy and IPAA formation which were comparable to the ones obtained with laparoscopic surgery [36]. The authors concluded that, when performed in a referral center, the positive results of laparoscopic surgery are unlikely to be improved by the robotic approach. Nevertheless, considering the continuous technical advancement, future studies might highlight the potential benefits of this procedure.

References

1. Guillou PJ, Quirke P, Thorpe H et al; MRC CLASICC trial group (2005) Short-term endpoints of conventional versus laparoscopic-assisted surgery in patients with colorectal cancer (MRC CLASICC trial): multicentre, randomised controlled trial. Lancet 365(9472):1718–1726
2. Clinical Outcomes of Surgical Therapy Study Group; Nelson H, Sargent DJ et al (2004) A comparison of laparoscopically assisted and open colectomy for colon cancer. N Engl J Med. 350(20):2050–2059
3. Schwenk W, Haase O, Neudecker J, Müller JM (2005) Short term benefits for laparoscopic colorectal resection. Cochrane Database Syst Rev 2005(3):CD003145
4. Targownik LE, Singh H, Nugent Z, Bernstein CN (2012) The epidemiology of colectomy in ulcerative colitis: results from a population-based cohort. Am J Gastroenterol 107(8):1228–1235
5. Filippi J, Allen PB, Hébuterne X, Peyrin-Biroulet L (2011) Does anti-TNF therapy reduce the requirement for surgery in ulcerative colitis? A systematic review. Curr Drug Targets 12(10):1440–1447

6. Ahmed Ali U, Keus F, Heikens JT et al (2009) Open versus laparoscopic (assisted) ileo pouch anal anastomosis for ulcerative colitis and familial adenomatous polyposis. Cochrane Database Syst Rev 2009(1):CD006267
7. Fleming FJ, Francone TD, Kim MJ et al (2011) A laparoscopic approach does reduce short-term complications in patients undergoing ileal pouch-anal anastomosis. Dis Colon Rectum 54(2):176–182
8. Bartels SA, D'Hoore A, Cuesta MA et al (2012) Significantly increased pregnancy rates after laparoscopic restorative proctocolectomy: a cross-sectional study. Ann Surg 256(6): 1045–1048
9. Beyer-Berjot L, Maggiori L, Birnbaum D et al (2013) A total laparoscopic approach reduces the infertility rate after ileal pouch-anal anastomosis: a 2-center study. Ann Surg 258(2):275–282
10. Øresland T, Bemelman WA, Sampietro GM et al; European Crohn's and Colitis Organisation (ECCO) (2015) European evidence based consensus on surgery for ulcerative colitis. J Crohns Colitis 9(1):4–25
11. Tekkis PP, Fazio VW, Lavery IC et al (2005) Evaluation of the learning curve in ileal pouch-anal anastomosis surgery. Ann Surg 241(2):262–268
12. Rencuzogullari A, Stocchi L, Costedio M et al (2017) Characteristics of learning curve in minimally invasive ileal pouch-anal anastomosis in a single institution. Surg Endosc 31(3):1083–1092
13. Kiely JM, Fazio VW, Remzi FH et al (2012) Pelvic sepsis after IPAA adversely affects function of the pouch and quality of life. Dis Colon Rectum 55(4):387–392
14. Gu J, Stocchi L, Remzi FH, Kiran RP (2014) Total abdominal colectomy for severe ulcerative colitis: does the laparoscopic approach really have benefit? Surg Endosc 28(2): 617–625
15. Causey MW, Stoddard D, Johnson EK et al (2013) Laparoscopy impacts outcomes favorably following colectomy for ulcerative colitis: a critical analysis of the ACS-NSQIP database. Surg Endosc 27(2):603–609
16. Greenstein AJ, Romanoff AM, Moskowitz AJ et al (2013) Payer status and access to laparoscopic subtotal colectomy for ulcerative colitis. Dis Colon Rectum 56(9):1062–1067
17. Fajardo AD, Dharmarajan S, George V et al (2010) Laparoscopic versus open 2-stage ileal pouch: laparoscopic approach allows for faster restoration of intestinal continuity. J Am Coll Surg 211(3):377–383
18. Bartels SA, Gardenbroek TJ, Ubbink DT et al (2013) Systematic review and meta-analysis of laparoscopic versus open colectomy with end ileostomy for non-toxic colitis. Br J Surg 100(6):726–733
19. Shapiro R, Vogel JD, Kiran RP (2011) Risk of postoperative venous thromboembolism after laparoscopic and open colorectal surgery: an additional benefit of the minimally invasive approach? Dis Colon Rectum 54(12):1496–1502
20. Stocchi L (2010) Laparoscopic surgery for ulcerative colitis. Clin Colon Rectal Surg 23(4):248–258
21. Rottoli M, Vallicelli C, Gionchetti P et al (2018) Transabdominal salvage surgery after pouch failure in a tertiary center: a case-matched study. Dig Liver Dis 50(5):446–451
22. Rottoli M, Vallicelli C, Bigonzi E et al (2018) Prepouch ileitis after ileal pouch-anal anastomosis: patterns of presentation and risk factors for failure of treatment. J Crohns Colitis 12(3):273–279
23. Brady RR, Collie MH, Ho GT et al (2008) Outcomes of the rectal remnant following colectomy for ulcerative colitis. Colorectal Dis 10(2):144–150
24. Longo WE (2013) The out-of-circuit rectum in ulcerative colitis: the bumpy road less traveled: comment on "Fate of rectal stump after subtotal colectomy for ulcerative colitis in the era of ileal pouch-anal anastomosis". JAMA Surg 148(5):412
25. Buchs NC, Mortensen NJ, Guy RJ, George BD (2016) Persistent colitis after emergency laparoscopic subtotal colectomy for ulcerative colitis: a cautionary note. Colorectal Dis 18(1):106–107

26. Gu J, Stocchi L, Remzi F, Kiran RP (2013) Intraperitoneal or subcutaneous: does location of the (colo)rectal stump influence outcomes after laparoscopic total abdominal colectomy for ulcerative colitis? Dis Colon Rectum 56(5):615–621

27. Karch LA, Bauer JJ, Gorfine SR, Gelernt IM (1995) Subtotal colectomy with Hartmann's pouch for inflammatory bowel disease. Dis Colon Rectum 38(6):635–639

28. Ito M, Sugito M, Kobayashi A et al (2008) Relationship between multiple numbers of stapler firings during rectal division and anastomotic leakage after laparoscopic rectal resection. Int J Colorectal Dis 23(7):703–707

29. Penna M, Hompes R, Arnold S et al; TaTME Registry Collaborative (2017) Transanal total mesorectal excision: international registry results of the first 720 cases. Ann Surg 266(1):111–117

30. Tasende MM, Delgado S, Jimenez M et al (2015) Minimal invasive surgery: NOSE and NOTES in ulcerative colitis. Surg Endosc 29(11):3313–3318

31. Liyanage C, Ramwell A, Harris GJ et al (2013) Transanal endoscopic microsurgery: a new technique for completion proctectomy. Colorectal Dis 15(9):e542–e547

32. de Buck van Overstraeten A, Mark-Christensen A, Wasmann KA et al (2017) Transanal versus transabdominal minimally invasive (completion) proctectomy with ileal pouch-anal anastomosis in ulcerative colitis: a comparative study. Ann Surg 266(5):878–883

33. Pedraza R, Patel CB, Ramos-Valadez DI, Haas EM (2011) Robotic-assisted laparoscopic surgery for restorative proctocolectomy with ileal J pouch-anal anastomosis. Minim Invasive Ther Allied Technol 20(4):234–239

34. McLemore EC, Cullen J, Horgan S et al (2012) Robotic-assisted laparoscopic stage II restorative proctectomy for toxic ulcerative colitis. Int J Med Robot 8(2):178–183

35. Miller AT, Berian JR, Rubin M et al (2012) Robotic-assisted proctectomy for inflammatory bowel disease: a case-matched comparison of laparoscopic and robotic technique. J Gastrointest Surg 16(3):587–594

36. Rencuzogullari A, Gorgun E, Costedio M et al (2016) Case-matched comparison of robotic versus laparoscopic proctectomy for inflammatory bowel disease. Surg Laparosc Endosc Percutan Tech 26(3):e37–e40

Results and Quality of Life after Surgical Treatment of Ulcerative Colitis

11

Gilberto Poggioli, Lorenzo Gentilini, Maurizio Coscia, and Federica Ugolini

11.1 Introduction

Restorative proctocolectomy and ileal pouch-anal anastomosis (IPAA) has become standard surgical therapy for patients with ulcerative colitis and familial adenomatous polyposis. This procedure is technically demanding and is carried out to improve the patient's quality of life (QoL) by maintaining transanal defecation and continence after complete removal of the diseased large bowel mucosa thus avoiding permanent ileostomy.

Ileal pouch-anal anastomosis has been shown to have low morbidity; complications occur in the first months after surgery and can frequently be treated without influencing pouch function and the patient's QoL [1]. Early pouch failure is a rare condition and occurs in fewer than 10% of patients after a 10-year follow-up [2]. The main factors associated with pouch failure are the onset of fistulas of the pouch (pouch-anal or pouch-vaginal), chronic pouchitis, pre-pouch ileitis, pelvic sepsis and delayed diagnosis of Crohn's disease. All these conditions if not properly treated could result in poor functional outcomes, requiring a pouch excision or a fecal diversion with a loop ileostomy [3, 4].

Patients with functioning IPAAs report good functional outcomes, a good QoL, and state high satisfaction with the surgery. A recent systematic review regarding QoL and functional results after IPAA showed that outcomes quickly improve during the first months after surgery, and they could be considered indistinguishable from the general population 12 months after restorative proctocolectomy [5].

L. Gentilini (✉)
General Surgery Unit, Department of Digestive Diseases, S. Orsola-Malpighi Hospital
Bologna, Italy
e-mail: lorenzo.gentilini@aosp.bo.it

G. Poggioli (Ed), *Ulcerative Colitis,*
Updates in Surgery
DOI: 10.1007/978-88-470-3977-3_11, © Springer-Verlag Italia 2019

According to the functional results, patients report a number of bowel movements in 24 hours which could range from 5–7, with 1–2 evacuations at night. Urgency is reported in 4–11% of patients and increases over time with aging of the patient or in the presence of episodes of pouchitis [1, 2]. Fecal incontinence is rarely reported by patients; fewer than 20% of patients report episodes of seepage or soiling, without changes in frequency in the first decade after surgery [2]. In a meta-analysis including more than 9000 patients, severe and mild fecal incontinence were reported in 3.7% and 17% of patients, respectively [1]. The presence of incontinence is associated with the need for protective pads; their use did not change during follow-up and was reported in 20% and 25% of patients during the day and at night, respectively, in a large cohort of patients at the Cleveland Clinic [2].

Quality of life after IPAA is generally excellent; the majority of patients have no dietary, work, social or sexual restrictions and report satisfactory health status with high energy levels and satisfaction with the surgery. These results have been reported worldwide from major, high-volume institutions [1, 2, 6]. Moreover, several studies have confirmed that QoL after IPAA is not influenced by the preoperative diagnosis. In fact, many studies have reported that more than 90% of patients were satisfied with the surgery and were happy with their decision to have IPAA, including those with a preoperative diagnosis of ulcerative colitis, Crohn's disease, familial polyposis or indeterminate colitis [1, 2].

Many factors can influence long-term functional outcomes and QoL after IPAA. Age at surgery and a longer follow-up; septic postoperative complications, surgical aspects (such as pouch design and type of pouch-anal anastomosis) and a change in histological diagnosis could modify pouch functions. Moreover, most patients are young and the impact of restorative proctocolectomy on sexual function must be carefully evaluated.

11.2   Functional Outcomes in Pediatric Patients

Pediatric patients undergo restorative proctocolectomy for the following three conditions: ulcerative colitis refractory to medical treatment, chronic ulcerative colitis with associated dysplasia or cancer or, more commonly, for prophylaxis for colonic cancer in polyposis. Prepubertal patients with ulcerative colitis could have significant growth retardation despite appropriate medical therapy; in all cases, surgery should be considered. Pediatric patients should initially undergo total abdominal colectomy with terminal ileostomy. Restorative proctectomy with IPAA must be performed after pubertal growth and the ileal pouch should be tailored to the body size of the patient in order to ensure better functional results. Following this indication, functional outcomes after surgery are good, and patients report a satisfactory QoL.

In 2013, Zmora and colleagues analyzed a cohort of 25 patients who had undergone restorative proctocolectomy with a preoperative diagnosis of ulcerative colitis. All patients had surgery at <18 years of age. The results obtained suggested that the functional outcomes among pediatric patients who undergo IPAA were better than the outcomes of adults [7]. These data were subsequently confirmed by Shannon in 2016. The authors analyzed a cohort of 74 patients treated with IPAA who had had a median age of 18 years at surgery. In this study, patients reported good functional outcome with a high rate of pouch retention at follow-up. All patients with a functioning IPAA had a satisfactory QoL. The authors concluded that IPAA was an excellent option for pediatric patients with ulcerative colitis, although not when the diagnosis was changed to Crohn's disease due to the development of fistulas which are risk factors for pouch failure [8].

Similar to adults, a J-pouch ileoanal anastomosis in pediatric patients is also associated with better functional results when compared to straight anastomosis without an ileal reservoir. Patients with a pouch have a consistently lower stool frequency and better continence rates [9].

Functional results and QoL improve over time in a pediatric cohort of patients. Michelassi reported a trend toward improved continence and reduced stool frequency over time, as did Nagar and Rabau, who described improved bowel movement frequency and nocturnal continence over time among pediatric patients [10, 11].

11.3 Functional Outcomes in Older Patients

Proctocolectomy with IPAA in the elderly is mainly performed for ulcerative colitis in patients refractory to maximal medical therapy or those dependent on high dose steroids, or in the presence of concomitant dysplasia or malignancy. Originally, the general consensus was that patients over 50 years of age should undergo proctocolectomy with formation of an end ileostomy due to the high morbidity associated with IPAA creation. Recently, several papers have documented similar outcomes with IPAA in terms of safety when compared to younger patients [12, 13]. A recent meta-analysis supports the view that in terms of safety, IPAA in patients over 50 years of age is feasible, with comparable complication rates to those seen in younger patients [14]. Different studies have advised that IPAA can be safely performed in older patients, even those in their 70s or 80s [15, 16].

A recent multicenter registry analysis undertaken by Cohan and colleagues which included 2493 patients undergoing IPAA with 254 over the age of 60, found that, in terms of postoperative complication rates, there was no significant increase in older patients; however, there was an increased length in hospital stay in the older group. The only difference in terms of postoperative complications according to age at surgery is an increased risk of dehydration and electrolyte imbalance reported in older patients (23.68% in younger patients versus 60% in those over 65). This was due to loop ileostomy in the early postoperative phase [13].

With regards to functional outcomes, some differences have been reported between younger and older patients. Data from a recent systematic review showed a significant difference in terms of incontinence rates, with older patients significantly more likely to suffer incontinence, both during the day and at night [14]. The number of bowel movements per 24 hours was statistically higher in patients over 50 years of age with minimal impact on overall daily living and QoL. Moreover, various papers have reported a deterioration in functional results with aging [14]. Patient satisfaction with the surgery and postoperative QoL remained high during follow-up, even in older patients [14].

The American Society of Colon and Rectal Surgeons recommends that chronological age should not be a reason in itself to deny IPAA in older patients [17]. Similarly, the ECCO guidelines state that there is no age limit for performing an IPAA as long the patient retains good anal sphincter function [18].

11.4   Changes in Functional Results over Time

An abundance of well-established data exists in the literature regarding short-term results after restorative proctocolectomy with IPAA. Functional results and QoL after surgery are good with high satisfaction for the surgical procedure in the first years after surgery.

The main long-term postoperative complications which can occur during follow-up are chronic pouchitis, pouch-anal or pouch vaginal fistulas and anastomotic strictures while pre-pouch ileitis is rare.

Chronic pouchitis is the most frequent long-term complication reported in many studies. The incidence of this condition increases over time and ranges from 20% to 40% of patients. Two large series of patients with follow-up shorter than 20 years have reported chronic pouchitis in at least 21% of patients undergoing IPAA [19, 20]. A study from the Cleveland Clinic has emphasized a significantly higher rate of pouchitis after 15 years, up to 39% [2], while chronic pouchitis has been diagnosed in 28.6% of patients with more than 20 years of follow-up in a single center retrospective study [21]. These heterogeneous data could be explained by the authors' use of a non-standard accepted definition of "pouchitis" and by the different lengths of follow-up in the various studies.

Similar to pouchitis, the onset of fistulizing disease is also related to the length of the follow-up. The incidence of pouch-anal or pouch-vaginal fistulas is low in patients with a short follow-up (less than 3%) and it increases to 10% in patients with follow-ups longer than 15 years [2, 22]; its incidence is even higher, up to 30%, in patients with follow-ups longer than 20 years [21].

Anastomotic stenosis is a frequent condition; its incidence remains stable over time and it ranges from 11% to 13% of patients in large series without differences according to the type of ileo-anal anastomosis [2, 20, 21]. Stenosis can easily be treated in many cases with self-dilation, with good compliance of the patient and a high healing rate. Stenosis rarely leads to pouch failure.

Finally, pre-pouch ileitis can occur in patients treated with restorative proctocolectomy over time; however, this condition is a rare long-term complication which occurs in fewer than 5–8% of patients [21, 23]. The pathogenesis of pre-pouch ileitis is unclear. Many studies have suggested a misdiagnosis of Crohn's disease; instead, some authors have proposed that pre-pouch ileitis may be the result of reflux of the pouch contents often associated with concomitant pouchitis. Pre-pouch ileitis frequently requires medical therapy; in cases of medical failure, patients should undergo endoscopic dilatation or surgical resection which is associated with a high risk of pouch failure.

Pouch failure results in complete pouch removal with a Brooke ileostomy or the fashioning of a diverting ileostomy (never reversed) without pouch removal. The pouch failure rate increases over time with lengthening of the follow-up. In a cohort of 3707 patients, Fazio et al. described a pouch failure rate of 5.3% after a mean follow-up of 15 years; 3.6% of the cases required excision of the pouch and 1.4% had redo IPAA, whereas 0.3% had a non-functioning pouch [2]. In other studies, having a follow-up of more than 20 years, the pouch failure rate was higher in up to 11% of cases [24, 25]. These data have been confirmed by a recent retrospective single center study involving a cohort of 185 patients treated for a preoperative diagnosis of ulcerative colitis with a mean follow-up of 24 years. In this group of patients, the pouch failure rate was 10.8%; the pouch retention rate decreased gradually over time without sudden changes until the end of the follow-up [21]. The main factors associated with pouch failure as reported by different authors were pelvic sepsis, the onset of pouch-anal and pouch-vaginal fistulas and a delayed diagnosis of Crohn's disease [21, 26, 27].

Similarly, to the onset of long-term postoperative complications functional results and QoL can also be influenced by the passage of time. Despite the considerable amount of data available regarding short-term outcomes, the number of studies specifically addressing changes in functional results over time is limited. Moreover, the few data reported in the literature are often conflicting; some authors assert that long-term functional outcomes are maintained over time [10, 19] while other studies describe a worsening of the functional results over time [22, 28].

Many studies have shown that IPAA confers good long-term functional results after an initial period of adjustment of 12–18 months, after which the frequency of bowel movements stabilizes at 6–7/day with good continence and the ability to postpone a bowel movement until convenient [10]. Subsequently, bowel movement frequency remains constant in the first decade after surgery without the need for dietary restriction and with a decrease in the use of antimotility drugs over time. According to these data, a systematic review by Heikens et al. conducted on more than 4000 patients concluded that QoL improves in the first 12 months after surgery and reaches results indistinguishable from the healthy population [5]. However, with the lengthening of the follow-up, functional results deteriorate. A recent study of the Cleveland Clinic Group conducted on a large cohort of 396 patients with a follow-up of more than a minimum of 15 years reported a significant increasing of bowel movements, urgency and incontinence 15 years after IPAA [22].

A similar trend in bowel movements has been reported by a Mayo Clinic study (1885 patients with a mean follow up of 10.8 years) which showed a slight deterioration in stool frequency during the day and at night. Moreover, they reported episodes of fecal incontinence, more frequent 10 years after surgery which remained relatively stable between 10 and 20 years [29]. A single-center retrospective study analyzing only patients with a follow-up of more than 20 years confirmed the deterioration of the functional results with the lengthening of the follow-up. The authors observed an increase in median bowel movements over time after surgery, which reached significance only for night-time evacuations. Urgency did not change after the primary surgery. However, the use of antimotility drugs, and the incidence of major and minor incontinence increased significantly after more than 20 years. The main reasons for this slight worsening of the functional results over time can be identified in the physiological aging of the population studied after such a long follow-up, or by the increase in incidence over years of pouchitis, as previously mentioned.

Despite this slight deterioration in function over time the QoL reported by the patients in different studies remains high. The subjective perceptions of the patients regarding their own QoL, energy and vitality did not show any changes after restorative proctocolectomy, with high scores reported throughout the follow-up. The majority of patients were willing to recommend an ileoanal pouch to others in a similar medical situation; patients who declared preference for a permanent stoma were rare [21, 24, 29, 30]. Some studies reported a deterioration in sexual function over years. However, this condition could be due to the aging of the study population; in fact, many studies conducted on a normal population of men and women showed a physiological decline in sexual desire and sexual activity over time.

11.5   Pelvic Sepsis after IPAA and Functional Results

Pelvic septic complications after restorative proctocolectomy such as pelvic abscess or anastomotic leak could negatively influence long-term functional results and QoL. The data reported in the literature are frequently conflicting regarding the effect of pelvic sepsis on functional outcomes. A study by Chessin et al. in 2008 evaluated the outcomes of 60 patients with an anastomotic leak after restorative proctocolectomy and reported that anastomotic leak did not adversely affect long-term QoL or functional outcomes [31]. Similarly, in their analysis Hallberg et al. reported that pelvic sepsis did not impair functional outcomes at long-term follow-up [32]. However, these studies suffered from the drawback of small numbers of patients with sepsis and the short duration of the follow-up.

Whereas some studies did not report impairment of long-term pouch functional outcomes after pelvic sepsis, other studies reported worse functional results in cases of pelvic abscess or anastomotic leak.

Farouk et al. analyzed a cohort of 1508 patients undergoing IPAA with 73 patients who developed pelvic septic complications. The authors reported that, in patients undergoing IPAA who developed a pelvic abscess, the abscess group had more daytime incontinence, required more medication to alter stool consistency or decrease frequency, and wore protective pads more often than those who did not develop abscesses [33]. Similar results were previously obtained by Breen in 1998. In this study conducted on 628 patients with IPAA with 41 cases of pelvic sepsis, a statistically significant increased number of bowel movements over a 24-hour period has been reported in those who developed pelvic sepsis (7.1 vs. 5.9; $p=0.009$). In addition, fewer of these patients also maintained the ability to differentiate between the passage of stool or gas from their pouch (50% vs. 77%, $p=0.02$) [34].

A worsening of functional results in patients with pelvic sepsis has been confirmed by a recent Cleveland Clinic study. This study, conducted in 2012 on a large cohort of more than 3000 patients with IPAA over a 24-year period, demonstrated that pelvic sepsis leads to impairment of both functional outcomes and QoL. The authors considered pelvic sepsis to be any infective process in the peripouch area detected by means of clinical evidence, including all abscesses associated with or without anastomotic leak and/or the formation of chronic perineal sinus with a cavity, or fistulas, detected by clinical or radiological means as opposed to pouch leak alone. Regarding functional outcomes, patients with septic complications had worse pouch function. The number of daytime, night-time, and total daily bowel movements was similar between patients with or without complications; however, those who developed sepsis reported significantly worse incontinence over the long term. Although pad usage during the day and night was similar in all patients, daytime seepage was significantly worse in patients with septic complications. More patients in the septic group also reported a higher incidence of urgency. Moreover, in this study, patients with pelvic sepsis who retained their pouch were more likely to experience some form of pouch dysfunction with a greater degree of dietary, social, sexual, and work-related restrictions, and some degree of impaired QoL. Finally, after septic complications, fewer patients were likely to recommend IPAA to others with their similar medical situation [35].

A recent population-based study reinforced the long-term deleterious effects of serious early complications on functional outcomes of restorative proctocolectomy with IPAA and provided additional motivation to minimize their occurrence. This study published in 2016 analyzed the effect of early postoperative complications in a cohort of 136 patients undergoing IPAA with a median follow-up of 12 years. Postoperative complications were classified according to the Clavien–Dindo scale. Patients who reported Clavien–Dindo grade 3 or 4 early complications had lower QoL scores when compared with uncomplicated patients [36].

The factors which contribute to a poorly functioning pouch as a result of pelvic sepsis are still not well understood. Many conditions due to pelvic inflammation have been considered by various authors. A narrowed anastomosis secondary to surrounding pelvic fibrosis, pouch dysmotility, impaired pelvic floor activity or fistula formation, and a fibrotic, poorly compliant pouch which does not retain stool adequately may be included among these. Finally, many studies have reported a higher risk of pouch failure for patients who developed pelvic sepsis after IPAA [36–38].

All patients with postoperative septic complications should be identified promptly and successfully treated in order to reduce the impact of pelvic inflammation on long-term functional results and to decrease the risk of pouch failure.

11.6 Pouch Design and Functional Results

Since the introduction of restorative proctocolectomy with IPAA, many pouch designs have been proposed. Currently, the most commonly used pouch design is the J-pouch which is easier and faster to fashion [39]. Other designs, such as S-, W- or K-pouches, have been described by different authors [40–42].

The S-pouch is the original design of the pouch proposed by Parks and Nicholls in 1978. It can be created using three limbs of 12–15 cm of terminal small bowel with a 2–3 cm exit conduit. This pouch must be hand-sewn without the use of staplers. Various studies have compared postoperative complications, functional outcomes, QoL, and pouch survival or failure rate between the S-pouch and the J-pouch. The majority of these studies did not find any differences in terms of postoperative complications or pouch failure rates, with similar functional results and QoL [43–45]. Some studies have described better continence of the S-pouch with subsequently better functional results with reduction of daily evacuations. However, the possible advantages of the S-pouch have been abrogated by frequently encountered difficulties with evacuation secondary to long efferent limbs, with up to 53% of patients having to catheterize their pouches. Combined with its more complex construction, this has led to a decline in the use of the S-pouch.

According to these data, a J-pouch is preferred to an S-pouch because it is more easily fashioned. A technical advantage of the S-pouch is the presence of a long efferent limb; therefore, this type of pouch is actually preferred when a J-pouch will not reach into the pelvis without tension, and a lengthening of the ileum is not possible or not sufficient. Moreover, a study published in 2015 demonstrated the superiority of the S design in patients undergoing a hand-sewn pouch-anal anastomosis. This study compared patients with J and S pouches with those having a hand-sewn pouch-anal anastomosis. The data obtained reported fewer postoperative complications and better functional results in patients having S pouches. Despite the fact that short-term complications in the 2 groups were similar, pouch fistula or sinus, pelvic sepsis, postoperative partial small-bowel obstruction, and postoperative pouch-related hospitalization occurred in fewer patients with an S-pouch. At a median follow-up of 12.2 years, patients with an S-pouch were found to have fewer bowel movements, less frequent pad use and a lower incidence of fecal incontinence. No differences in pouch failure rate were described by the authors [46]. According to these findings, an S-pouch should be considered in cases of hand-sewn pouch-anal anastomosis in order to reach the pelvic floor without tension and with better long-term functional results.

The W-pouch was proposed by Nicholls and Pezim in 1985. They described the potential advantages of this type of pouch, namely a lower number of bowel movements during the day and at night, and no requirement for pouch intubation. Subsequently, various authors compared the J-and the W-pouches on the basis of functional results. Four randomized controlled trials have been published comparing J- and W-pouches. Two trials, one of 60 and one of 33 patients, showed no difference in function between J- and W-pouches at up to 12 months of follow-up [47, 48]. Another two trials of 24 and 50 patients showed a mean daily defecation frequency higher in patients treated with a J-pouch, associated with increased use of antimotility drugs [49, 50]. The functional advantages of the W-pouch could be due to its greater volume, allowing in theory for improved reservoir capacity, thus reducing defecation frequency and incontinence episodes. Despite the few advantages of a W-pouch reported by some authors, their use is not currently diffuse due to higher technical difficulties in their fashioning; this procedure is more time-consuming because it has to be hand-sewn without the use of staplers. Moreover, the bulkiness of a W-pouch may also result in greater difficulty in placing the pouch into a narrow pelvis. Finally, a randomized controlled trial conducted in 2012 suggested that the theoretical functional advantage of the W-pouch due to its greater volume exists only in the short term and is of little consequence to the patient's long-term QoL. The authors evaluated 94 patients randomly assigned to J- or W-pouches and assessed functional outcomes at 1 and 9 years after surgery. At 1 year, there was a significant difference in 24-hour bowel movement, with a higher frequency of daytime evacuation in J- vs. W-pouches, but with no difference in nocturnal function. At the 9-year follow-up, function had equalized between the two groups, with no differences in bowel movements either during the day or at night. The authors concluded that, currently, the J-pouch should be considered the ideal pouch design because it has been clearly shown to be easier to construct while having minimal functional disadvantages, which are attenuated over time and which have no significant impact on the patient's QoL [51].

The relatively little influence of pouch design on functional results has also been confirmed by a large meta-analysis carried out in 2007. This analysis involved 18 studies with 1519 patients (689 J-pouches, 306 W-pouches and 524 S-pouches) and did not detect any significant differences in early postoperative complications including leak, stricture, pelvic sepsis, pouchitis, small bowel obstruction and pouch failure. The data obtained demonstrated a higher frequency of bowel movements in patients with a J-pouch than those treated with either S-or W-pouches. However, patients with S- or W-pouches were more likely to experience obstructed evacuation and frequently required the use of enemas or intubation. Seepage and incontinence were similar among the three types of pouch designs [43].

The remaining pouch designs have not been completely validated by published studies and have not reached widespread diffusion in clinical practice. Of these remaining designs, some authors have suggested the use of the K-pouch.

A recent study conducted in 2016 on 103 patients who underwent restorative proctocolectomy with J- or K-pouches analyzed the differences between these two pouch designs. No patients in either group have had their pouch removed or defunctioned due to failure at a mean follow-up of 8 years, and no significant differences were reported by the authors in overall pouch functional scores between patients treated with a J-pouch or a K-pouch, although there was a non-significant tendency towards better function in the latter [52].

Similarly, a prospective randomized comparison by Øresland et al. in 1990 found a non-significant tendency to better functional outcome in patients treated with a K-pouch when compared to a J-pouch [53]. Conversely, in a non-randomized study on 412 IPAAs presented by Bloc et al. in 2009, patients with a K-pouch reported better long-term functional results as compared with outcomes described by patients with a J-pouch [54]. Probably the fewer advantages reported by patients with K-pouches could be due to the larger pouch volume with the same length of ileum used with subsequent greater continence of the pouch itself. Despite these advantages, K-pouch construction is somewhat more complicated, requiring both hand suturing rather than stapling and increased operative time. Moreover, the complexity of this procedure requires a specialized unit with experienced surgeons; therefore, the J-pouch design is currently preferred.

In conclusion, the J-pouch design is currently the most used in the world due to its technically easier creation associated with good functional results without the need for pouch intubation and is preferred by more than 95% of surgeons worldwide.

11.7   Functional Outcomes According to Type of Pouch Anal Anastomosis

Since the introduction of restorative proctocolectomy, two types of IPAA have been described. A hand-sewn anastomosis can be performed with mucosectomy of the rectal stump followed by hand suturing between the ileal pouch and the anal canal. Mucosectomy has the advantage of removing the diseased bowel mucosa, particularly if taken down to the dentate line; this is preferred in patients with familial adenomatous polyposis or ulcerative colitis in the presence of dysplasia. The alternative technique is to retain the mucosa of the rectal stump and perform a stapled pouch-anal anastomosis. This technique is quicker and easier to perform, and it involves less manipulation of the anal canal, therefore reducing the risk of postoperative problems with continence. However, a stapled anastomosis leaves potentially diseased and possibly inflamed rectal mucosa which requires regular follow-up of the anal transition zone due to the risk of dysplasia and cancer.

Various authors have compared hand-sewn and stapled anastomoses according to functional results and QoL.

Two different meta-analyses were published in 2006 comparing these two types of anastomosis. The meta-analysis by Schluender et al., which included four prospective randomized trials, analyzed 180 patients with a preoperative diagnosis of ulcerative colitis and familial adenomatous polyposis. This study demonstrated that there were no significant differences in functional outcomes between hand-sewn and stapled IPAAs [55]. Conversely, the second meta-analysis presented by Lovegrove et al. evaluated 4183 patients who underwent restorative proctocolectomy with a preoperative diagnosis of ulcerative colitis or familial adenomatous polyposis (2699 hand-sewn vs. 1484 stapled anastomoses). The data obtained showed a superiority of stapled anastomoses in functional results, in particular regarding continence. In fact, patients with a hand-sewn anastomosis had a higher rate of seepage at night together with incontinence of liquid stool with subsequent increased use of protective pads at night. The two techniques were similar with regard to stool frequency per 24 h defecation at night and use of antidiarrheal medication. Similarly, no differences were reported in the onset of early postoperative complications such as anastomotic leak, pelvic sepsis, pouch-related fistula, pouchitis, anastomotic stricture and pouch failure [56].

In 2009, Kirat et al. presented a large retrospective study by a single institution comparing 2270 stapled and 474 hand-sewn anastomoses. The data obtained were similar to those already reported by Lovegrove et al. A stapled IPAA had better outcomes and QoL compared with those with a hand-sewn anastomosis; this type of anastomosis was associated with lower frequency of incontinence, seepage and pad usage with subsequent reduction in dietary, social and work restrictions. Moreover, postoperative complications such as anastomotic stricture, septic complications, bowel obstruction and pouch failure, were also significantly fewer among the patients who received a stapled anastomosis [57].

A higher risk of postoperative complications in patients with a hand-sewn anastomosis has also been reported in a recent study by the Cleveland Clinic. In 2013, Fazio et al. published the results of a large retrospective study conducted on 3707 patients treated with IPAA at their institution. Comparing patients undergoing hand-sewn or stapled anastomoses, they observed a higher rate of anastomotic leak in the hand-sewn group (9.21% vs. 6.06%, p=0.009). Similarly, the rates of postoperative hemorrhage (6.9% vs. 3.83%, p=0.002), anastomotic stricture (23.03% vs. 15.29%, p=0.001), pouch fistulas (12.67% vs. 8.47%, p=0.002) and obstruction (22.65% vs. 17.14%, p=0.003) were higher in patients undergoing a hand-sewn pouch-anal anastomosis. Pouch failure rate (12.09% vs. 4.21%, p=0.0001) and the need for redo IPAA (12.28% vs 4.21%, p=0.001) were also higher in the hand-sewn group [2].

Poorer functional results in patients with a hand-sewn anastomosis can be due to the manipulation of the anal canal with risk of damage to the sphincter mechanism and subsequent alteration in anal sphincter pressure. Moreover, the mucosa of the anal transition zone has a rich sensory innervation, which is involved in differentiating between flatus and stool; its removal performed during mucosectomy could contribute to the worsening of functional outcomes with the onset of incontinence.

Currently, a stapled IPAA is the preferred technique because it is easier and quicker to perform and is associated with better long-term functional outcomes. A hand-sewn anastomosis is preferred in patients with a failure of the stapled technique or in patients requiring redo surgery.

11.8   Functional Outcomes in Patients with Crohn's Disease

Restorative proctocolectomy is the treatment of choice for patients with a preoperative diagnosis of ulcerative colitis or familial adenomatous polyposis; however, an ileal pouch could also be fashioned in patients with Crohn's colitis.

Patients with Crohn's colitis and rectal sparing usually undergo total abdominal colectomy with ileorectal anastomosis. Patients with severe proctitis refractory to medical therapy cannot be treated with ileorectal anastomosis and should undergo proctectomy; in these patients, an IPAA could be attempted to avoid permanent ileostomy. Restorative proctocolectomy can be performed intentionally in patients with Crohn's proctocolitis but only in highly selected cases without ileal or perianal involvement. Functional results, QoL and pouch failure rate in these highly selected patients intentionally undergoing IPAA are satisfactory and similar to patients with a preoperative diagnosis of ulcerative colitis [58].

Crohn's disease can also be found inadvertently in the colectomy specimens of patients with a preoperative diagnosis of ulcerative colitis (incidental diagnosis) or it could develop de novo in patients with a preoperative diagnosis of ulcerative colitis and without evidence of Crohn's disease on the surgical specimen (delayed diagnosis).

A recent Cleveland Clinic study compared functional outcomes and QoL in patients undergoing IPAA with an intentional, incidental or delayed diagnosis of Crohn's disease. The data obtained reported a higher pouch retention rate in patients intentionally or incidentally treated with IPAA when compared with patients having delayed diagnosis of Crohn's disease. Patients with a delayed diagnosis of Crohn have higher rates of pouch-anal and pouch-vaginal fistulas, chronic pouchitis and anastomotic strictures with subsequent higher rates of pouch failure. Moreover, patients with an intentional or an incidental diagnosis of Crohn's disease had a better score in functional outcome evaluation [59].

A higher risk of pouch failure and postoperative complications has been confirmed for patients with Crohn's disease by a Cleveland Clinic study. In this study, 2953 IPAAs for ulcerative colitis were compared to 63 and 150 pouches for indeterminate colitis and Crohn's disease, respectively.

Pouch fistulas were observed in a total of 158 patients; the incidence of fistulas was similar between the histological subgroups within the first 90 days, but late fistulas were significantly more likely among patients with Crohn's disease than among other histological subgroups (odds ratio: 3.16, $p=0.001$). Similarly, patients with Crohn's disease were more likely to develop pouch failure than other diagnoses ($p<0.001$). Specifically, patients with Crohn's disease were 2.85 times and 3.08 times more likely to develop pouch failure than those with mucosal ulcerative colitis and indeterminate colitis, respectively [2]. In patients who retained their pouch, overall functional outcomes and QoL were similar for mucosal ulcerative colitis when compared with familial adenomatous polyposis, Crohn's disease, and indeterminate colitis [2].

11.9   Restorative Proctocolectomy and Sexual Function

The majority of patients undergoing IPAA are young; therefore, sexual function is an important aspect which should be carefully evaluated.

Several studies have concluded that sexual function remains relatively unchanged postoperatively after restorative proctocolectomy [60, 61]. Some authors have suggested that sexual function may even improve after surgery [62]. A possible reason for this improvement in sexual function is that patients with inflammatory bowel disease with colon and rectum in situ are more likely than the average population to have reduced sexual function, and the tendency is stronger in patients with active disease than in patients in remission. After surgery, these patients could present an improvement in general health due to better stool control with subsequent benefit in sexual function. Data from the literature have reported adequate sexual functioning which remains stable over a relatively short postoperative follow-up period in patients who undergo surgery during adulthood [61–64].

However, restorative proctocolectomy with IPAA, as in any form of pelvic surgery has the risk of altering sexual function. The impact of IPAA on sexual function is probably multifactorial. The proctectomy could lead to pelvic nerve damage resulting in retrograde ejaculation and impotence in men, and vaginal dryness in women, leading to reduced sexual function. In addition, anatomical changes as a result of the surgery can lead to vaginal adhesions in women resulting in dyspareunia. The rates of sexual erectile dysfunction and retrograde ejaculation in men range from 0% to 25% after surgery [61], while dyspareunia varies from 22% to 30% [63]. Sexual dysfunction is not always reported by the patient during follow-up; this could justify such a varied incidence of sexual dysfunction as reported by various studies.

Postoperative functional outcomes can also negatively affect sexual function. Patients with poor pouch function could report poor sexual function postoperatively. The impact of poor pouch function on sexual activity seems to be higher in female patients. A recent study did not find a significant correlation between impaired sexual function and poor pouch function in men having undergone pouch surgery while women had a significant correlation between impaired sexual function and poor pouch function [65].

References

1. Hueting WE, Buskens E, van der Tweel I et al (2005) Results and complications after ileal pouch anal anastomosis: a meta-analysis of 43 observational studies comprising 9,317 patients. Dig Surg 22(1–2):69–79
2. Fazio VW, Kiran RP, Remzi FH et al (2013) Ileal pouch anal anastomosis: analysis of outcome and quality of life in 3707 patients. Ann Surg 257(4):679–685
3. Grucela AL, Bauer JJ, Gorfine SR, Chessin DB (2011) Outcome and long-term function of restorative proctocolectomy for Crohn's disease: comparison to patients with ulcerative colitis. Colorectal Dis 13(4):426–430
4. Shen B, Patel S, Lian L (2010) Natural history of Crohn's disease in patients who underwent intentional restorative proctocolectomy with ileal pouch-anal anastomosis. Aliment Pharmacol Ther 31(7):745–753
5. Heikens JT, de Vries J, van Laarhoven CJ (2012) Quality of life, health-related quality of life and health status in patients having restorative proctocolectomy with ileal pouch-anal anastomosis for ulcerative colitis: a systematic review. Colorectal Dis 14(5):536–544
6. Tekkis PP, Lovegrove RE, Tilney HS et al (2010) Long-term failure and function after restorative proctocolectomy – a multi-centre study of patients from the UK National Ileal Pouch Registry. Colorectal Dis 12(5):433–441
7. Zmora O, Natanson M, Dotan I et al (2013) Long-term functional and quality-of-life outcomes after IPAA in children. Dis Colon Rectum 56(2):198–204

8. Shannon A, Eng K, Kay M et al (2016) Long-term follow up of ileal pouch anal anastomosis in a large cohort of pediatric and young adult patients with ulcerative colitis. J Pediatr Surg 51(7):1181–1186
9. Seetharamaiah R, West BT, Ignash SJ et al (2009) Outcomes in pediatric patients undergoing straight vs J pouch ileoanal anastomosis: a multicenter analysis. J Pediatr Surg 44(7):1410–1417
10. Michelassi F, Lee J, Rubin M et al (2003) Long-term functional results after ileal pouch anal restorative proctocolectomy for ulcerative colitis: a prospective observational study. Ann Surg 238(3):433–441; discussion 442–445
11. Nagar H, Rabau M (2000) The importance of early surgery in children with ulcerative colitis. Isr Med Assoc J 2(8):592–594
12. Pellino G, Sciaudone G, Candilio G et al (2013) Complications and functional outcomes of restorative proctocolectomy for ulcerative colitis in the elderly. BMC Surg 13(Suppl 2):S9
13. Cohan JN, Bacchetti P, Varma MG, Finlayson E (2015) Outcomes after ileoanal pouch surgery in frail and older adults. J Surg Res 198(2):327–333
14. Ramage L, Qiu S, Georgiou P et al (2016) Functional outcomes following ileal pouch-anal anastomosis (IPAA) in older patients: a systematic review. Int J Colorectal Dis 31(3):481–492
15. Delaney CP, Dadvand B, Remzi FH et al (2002) Functional outcome, quality of life, and complications after ileal pouch-anal anastomosis in selected septuagenarians. Dis Colon Rectum 45(7):890–894; discussion 894
16. Pellino G, Sciaudone G, Candilio G et al (2014) Restorative proctocolectomy with ileal pouch-anal anastomosis is safe and effective in selected very elderly patients suffering from ulcerative colitis. Int J Surg 12(Suppl 2):S56–S59
17. Cohen JL, Strong SA, Hyman NH et al; Standards Practice Task Force American Society of Colon and Rectal Surgeons (2005) Practice parameters for the surgical treatment of ulcerative colitis. Dis Colon Rectum 48(11):1997–2009
18. Magro F, Gionchetti P, Eliakim R et al; European Crohn's and Colitis Organisation [ECCO] (2017) Third European evidence-based consensus on diagnosis and management of ulcerative colitis. Part 1: definitions, diagnosis, extra-intestinal manifestations, pregnancy, cancer surveillance, surgery, and ileo-anal pouch disorders. J Crohns Colitis 11(6):649–670
19. Karlbom U, Lindfors A, Påhlman L (2012) Long-term functional outcome after restorative proctocolectomy in patients with ulcerative colitis. Colorectal Dis 14(8):977–984
20. Rickard MJFX, Young CJ, Bissett IP et al; Research Committee of the Colorectal Surgical Society of Australasia (2007) Ileal pouch-anal anastomosis: the Australasian experience. Colorectal Dis 9(2):139–145
21. Gentilini L, Coscia M, Lombardi PM et al (2016) Ileal pouch-anal anastomosis 20 years later: is it still a good surgical option for patients with ulcerative colitis? Int J Colorectal Dis 31(12):1835–1843
22. Kiran RP, El-Gazzaz G, Remzi FH et al (2011) Influence of age at ileoanal pouch creation on long-term changes in functional outcomes. Colorectal Dis 13(2):184–190
23. McLaughlin SD, Clark SK, Bell AJ et al (2009) Incidence and short-term implications of prepouch ileitis following restorative proctocolectomy with ileal pouch-anal anastomosis for ulcerative colitis. Dis Colon Rectum 52(5):879–883
24. Berndtsson I, Lindholm E, Øresland T, Börjesson L (2007) Long-term outcome after ileal pouch-anal anastomosis: function and health-related quality of life. Dis Colon Rectum 50(10):1545–1552
25. Braveman JM, Schoetz DJ Jr, Marcello PW et al (2004) The fate of the ileal pouch in patients developing Crohn's disease. Dis Colon Rectum 47(10):1613–1619
26. Heuschen UA, Allemeyer EH, Hinz U et al (2002) Outcome after septic complications in J pouch procedures. Br J Surg 89(2):194–200
27. Ferrante M, Declerck S, De Hertogh G et al (2008) Outcome after proctocolectomy with ileal pouch-anal anastomosis for ulcerative colitis. Inflamm Bowel Dis 14(1):20–28

28. Tulchinsky H, Hawley PR, Nicholls J (2003) Long-term failure after restorative proctocolectomy for ulcerative colitis. Ann Surg 238(2):229–234
29. Hahnloser D, Pemberton JH, Wolff BG et al (2007) Results at up to 20 years after ileal pouch-anal anastomosis for chronic ulcerative colitis. Br J Surg 94(3):333–340
30. Bengtsson J, Börjesson L, Lundstam U, Øresland T (2007) Long-term function and manovolumetric characteristics after ileal pouch-anal anastomosis for ulcerative colitis. Br J Surg 94(3):327–332
31. Chessin DB, Gorfine SR, Bub DS et al (2008) Septic complications after restorative proctocolectomy do not impair functional outcome: long-term follow-up from a specialty center. Dis Colon Rectum 51(9):1312–1317
32. Hallberg H, Ståhlberg D, Akerlund JE (2005) Ileal pouch-anal anastomosis (IPAA): functional outcome after postoperative pelvic sepsis. A prospective study of 100 patients. Int J Colorectal Dis 20(6):529–533
33. Farouk R, Dozois RR, Pemberton JH, Larson D (1998) Incidence and subsequent impact of pelvic abscess after ileal pouch-anal anastomosis for chronic ulcerative colitis. Dis Colon Rectum 41(10):1239–1243
34. Breen EM, Schoetz DJ Jr, Marcello PW et al (1998) Functional results after perineal complications of ileal pouch-anal anastomosis. Dis Colon Rectum 41(6):691–695
35. Kiely JM, Fazio VW, Remzi FH et al (2012) Pelvic sepsis after IPAA adversely affects function of the pouch and quality of life. Dis Colon Rectum 55(4):387–392
36. McCombie A, Lee Y, Vanamala R et al (2016) Early postoperative complications have long-term impact on quality of life after restorative proctocolectomy. Medicine (Baltimore) 95(27):e3966
37. Forbes SS, O'Connor BI, Victor JC et al (2009) Sepsis is a major predictor of failure after ileal pouch-anal anastomosis. Dis Colon Rectum 52(12):1975–1981
38. Scott NA, Dozois RR, Beart RW et al (1988) Postoperative intra-abdominal and pelvic sepsis complicating ileal pouch-anal anastomosis. Int J Colorect Dis 3(3):149–152
39. Utsunomiya J, Iwama T, Imajo M et al (1980) Total colectomy, mucosal proctectomy, and ileoanal anastomosis. Dis Colon Rectum 23(7):459–466
40. Parks AG, Nicholls RJ (1978) Proctocolectomy without ileostomy for ulcerative colitis. Br Med J 2(6130):85–88
41. Nicholls RJ, Pezim ME (1985) Restorative proctocolectomy with ileal reservoir for ulcerative colitis and familial adenomatous polyposis: a comparison of three reservoir designs. Br J Surg 72(6):470–474
42. Hallgren T, Fasth S, Nordgren S et al (1989) Manovolumetric characteristics and functional results in three different pelvic pouch designs. Int J Colorectal Dis 4(3):156–160
43. Lovegrove RE, Heriot AG, Constantinides V et al (2007) Meta-analysis of short-term and long-term outcomes of J, W and S ileal reservoirs for restorative proctocolectomy. Colorectal Dis 9(4):310–320
44. McHugh SM, Diamant NE, McLeod R, Cohen Z (1987) S-pouches vs. J-pouches. A comparison of functional outcomes. Dis Colon Rectum 30(9):671–677
45. Tuckson WB, Fazio VW (1991) Functional comparison between double and triple ileal loop pouches. Dis Colon Rectum 34(1):17–21
46. Wu XR, Kirat HT, Kalady MF, Church JM (2015) Restorative proctocolectomy with a handsewn IPAA: S-pouch or J-pouch? Dis Colon Rectum 58(2):205–213
47. Johnston D, Williamson ME, Lewis WG et al (1996) Prospective controlled trial of duplicated (J) versus quadruplicated (W) pelvic ileal reservoirs in restorative proctocolectomy for ulcerative colitis. Gut 39(2):242–247
48. Keighley MR, Yoshioka K, Kmiot W (1988) Prospective randomized trial to compare the stapled double lumen pouch and the sutured quadruple pouch for restorative proctocolectomy. Br J Surg 75(10):1008–1011
49. Selvaggi F, Giuliani A, Gallo C et al (2000) Randomized, controlled trial to compare the J-pouch and W-pouch configurations for ulcerative colitis in the maturation period. Dis Colon Rectum 43(5):615–620

50. Lumley J, Stevenson A, Stitz R (2002) Prospective randomized study of J vs. W pouches in ulcerative colitis. Dis Colon Rectum 45:A5
51. McCormick PH, Guest GD, Clark AJ et al (2012) The ideal ileal-pouch design: a long-term randomized control trial of J- vs W-pouch construction. Dis Colon Rectum 55(12):1251–1257
52. Sunde ML, Øresland T, Faerden AE (2017) Restorative proctocolectomy with two different pouch designs: few complications with good function. Colorectal Dis 19(4):363–371
53. Øresland T, Fasth S, Nordgren S et al (1990) A prospective randomized comparison of two different pelvic pouch designs. Scand J Gastroenterol 25(10):986–996
54. Block M, Börjesson L, Lindholm E, Øresland T (2009) Pouch design and long-term functional outcome after ileal pouch-anal anastomosis. Br J Surg 96(5):527–532
55. Schluender SJ, Mei L, Yang H, Fleshner PR (2006) Can a meta-analysis answer the question: is mucosectomy and handsewn or double-stapled anastomosis better in ileal pouch-anal anastomosis? Am Surg 72(10):912–916
56. Lovegrove RE, Constantinides VA, Heriot AG et al (2006) A comparison of hand-sewn versus stapled ileal pouch anal anastomosis (IPAA) following proctocolectomy: a meta-analysis of 4183 patients. Ann Surg 244(1):18–26
57. Kirat HT, Remzi FH, Kiran RP, Fazio VW (2009) Comparison of outcomes after hand-sewn versus stapled ileal pouch-anal anastomosis in 3,109 patients. Surgery 146(4):723–729; discussion 729–730
58. Panis Y, Poupard B, Nemeth J et al (1996) Ileal pouch/anal anastomosis for Crohn's disease. Lancet 347(9005):854–857
59. Melton GB, Fazio VW, Kiran RP et al (2008) Long-term outcomes with ileal pouch-anal anastomosis and Crohn's disease: pouch retention and implications of delayed diagnosis. Ann Surg 248(4):608–616
60. Davies RJ, O'Connor BI, Victor C et al (2008) A prospective evaluation of sexual function and quality of life after ileal pouch-anal anastomosis. Dis Colon Rectum 51(7):1032–1035
61. Berndtsson I, Øresland T, Hultén L (2004) Sexuality in patients with ulcerative colitis before and after restorative proctocolectomy: a prospective study. Scand J Gastroenterol 39(4):374–379
62. Farouk R, Pemberton JH, Wolff BG et al (2000) Functional outcomes after ileal pouch-anal anastomosis for chronic ulcerative colitis. Ann Surg 231(6):919–926
63. Hueting WE, Gooszen HG, van Laarhoven CJ (2004) Sexual function and continence after ileo pouch anal anastomosis: a comparison between a meta-analysis and a questionnaire survey. Int J Colorectal Dis 19(3):215–218
64. Larson DW, Davies MM, Dozois EJ et al (2008) Sexual function, body image, and quality of life after laparoscopic and open ileal pouch-anal anastomosis. Dis Colon Rectum 51(4):392–396
65. Sunde ML, Øresland T, Færden AE (2016) Correlation between pouch function and sexual function in patients with IPAA. Scand J Gastroenterol 51(3):295–303

Long-term Complications after Surgical Treatment of Ulcerative Colitis

12

Gilberto Poggioli, Lorenzo Gentilini, Maurizio Coscia, and Federica Ugolini

12.1 Introduction

Patients undergoing restorative proctocolectomy with ileal pouch-anal anastomosis (IPAA) for ulcerative colitis (UC) could develop a wide range of long-term postoperative complications during their lifetime. These complications could negatively influence pouch function with a significant impact on the functional outcomes and quality of life of patients with IPAA. The main complications include: perianal fistulas (pouch-anal and pouch-vaginal fistulas), acute and chronic pouchitis, pre-pouch ileitis, cuffitis, anastomotic stenosis, Crohn's disease (CD) of the pouch, irritable pouch syndrome and mega-pouch. All these conditions are still a therapeutic challenge and require both medical and surgical treatment. Moreover, an unhealed complication could lead to pouch failure; therefore, careful treatment is required.

All complications are treated below, with the exception of pouch fistulas which will be treated in chapter 13.

12.2 Pouchitis

Pouchitis is the most frequent long-term complication of IPAA represented by non-specific inflammation of the ileal reservoir, resulting in variable clinical symptoms. Its occurrence is related to the duration of the follow-up and increases over time ranging from 5% to 50%; it occurs in up to 50% of patients 10 years after restorative proctocolectomy [1–3].

L. Gentilini (✉)
General Surgery Unit, Department of Digestive Diseases, S. Orsola-Malpighi Hospital
Bologna, Italy
e-mail: lorenzo.gentilini@aosp.bo.it

The incidence of this inflammatory complication is higher in patients treated with IPAA for UC than in patients with familial adenomatous polyposis; the reasons for the higher frequency of pouchitis in UC patients are still unknown.

In patients with familial adenomatous polyposis the cumulative incidence of pouchitis is much lower, ranging from 0% to 10%. Moreover, whether pouchitis develops more commonly within the initial years after IPAA or whether the risk increases continuously with follow-up remains undefined.

The etiology and pathogenesis of pouchitis are not entirely clear, and long-term management has been difficult. Risk factors, genetic associations, and serological markers of pouchitis suggest that close interaction between the host immune response and the pouch microbiota plays a relevant role in the etiology of this idiopathic inflammatory condition [4]. Fecal stasis and/or bacterial overgrowth in association with an abnormal mucosal immune response to altered commensal flora (dysbiosis) could lead to inflammation of the pouch. Some cases of pouchitis can be secondary to other conditions, such as infection from intestinal pathogens (*Clostridium difficile*, candida or cytomegalovirus) chronic use of nonsteroidal anti-inflammatory drugs (NSAIDs), current autoimmune disorders (celiac disease) or pouch ischemia.

The main risk factors for idiopathic pouchitis can be divided into genetic factors, disease related factors, preoperative status and postoperative conditions. The reported risk factors for pouchitis include genetic polymorphisms of the IL-1 receptor antagonist, non-carrier status of TNF allele 2 and NOD2/CARD15, extensive UC or colitis starting beyond the splenic flexure, backwash ileitis, preoperative corticosteroid or cyclosporine use, extraintestinal manifestations (especially arthropathy), thrombocytosis, being a non-smoker and the regular use of NSAIDs [5–8]. Similar to irritable bowel syndrome, visceral hypersensitivity has been described in these patients.

Pouchitis is not a homogenous disease entity; it can be represented by a wide spectrum of clinical presentations, endoscopic and histologic features, and disease courses and prognoses. The symptoms related to pouchitis include increased stool frequency, urgency, abdominal cramping, incontinence, nocturnal seepage, tenesmus, pelvic discomfort and arthralgia [9]. Rectal bleeding, fever and weight loss may also occur. The complications of pouchitis include abscesses, fistulas, stenosis of the pouch-anal anastomosis and adenocarcinoma of the pouch. No correlations have been found between the severity of the symptoms, and the degree of endoscopic or histologic inflammation of the pouch [10]. These symptoms are not all specific for pouchitis as they can also be reported by patients with other inflammatory or functional disorders of the pouch, such as cuffitis, CD of the pouch and irritable pouch syndrome. For this reason, a combined assessment of symptoms, and the endoscopic and histologic features should be carried out in order to diagnose pouchitis.

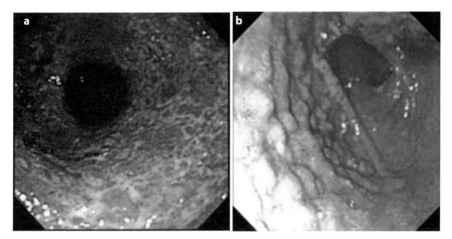

Fig. 12.1 Pouchitis at endoscopy

The main endoscopic findings compatible with pouchitis are diffuse erythema, edema, granularity, friability, spontaneous or contact bleeding, loss of vascular pattern, mucous exudates, hemorrhage, erosions and ulceration (Fig. 12.1). Endoscopy is also helpful in excluding other complications of the pouch, such as pre-pouch ileitis, cuffitis or CD of the pouch. Biopsies should be taken during a pouchoscopy to confirm the diagnosis and for surveillance for dysplasia.

The histologic features of acute inflammatory changes include ulceration, neutrophil infiltration and crypt abscess. Chronic histologic changes are villous blunting, hyperplasia of the crypt cells and an increased number of mononuclear cells in the lamina propria. The main aims of histological evaluation in clinical practice are the detection of specific pathogens (such as cytomegalovirus, candida and *C. difficile*), identification of ischemia and finding dysplasia.

For the purpose of research and clinical practice, various diagnostic criteria have been used. The most commonly used score is the "pouchitis disease activity index" (PDAI) developed at the Mayo Clinic, based on symptoms and endoscopic assessment with histological evaluation (Table 12.1) [9].

The PDAI provides a useful guide to abnormal findings and is the most commonly used instrument. An overall PDAI score is simple to calculate from three separate categories: clinical symptoms, endoscopic findings and histological changes. A total score of 7 or higher is defined as pouchitis.

In 2003, Shen et al. simplified the PDAI score in clinical practice with the introduction of the modified PDAI (mPDAI). This score is based only on clinical symptoms and endoscopic findings without data regarding the histologic features [11].

Table 12.1 Pouchitis disease activity index (PDAI) score

Criteria	Score
Clinical	
Stool frequency	
Usual postoperative stool frequency	0
1–2 stools/day > postoperative usual	1
3 or more stools/day > postoperative usual	2
Rectal bleeding	
None or rare	0
Present daily	1
Fecal urgency or abdominal cramps	
None	0
Occasional	1
Usual	2
Fever (temperature > 37.8° C)	
Absent	0
Present	1
Endoscopic inflammation	
Edema	0 / 1
Granularity	0 / 1
Friability	0 / 1
Loss of vascular pattern	0 / 1
Mucous exudates	0 / 1
Ulceration	0 / 1
Acute histologic inflammation	
Polymorphic nuclear leukocyte infiltration	
Mild	1
Moderate crypt abscess	2
Severe crypt abscess	3
Ulceration per low-power field (mean)	
<25%	1
25–50%	2
>50%	3

Pouchitis is defined as a PDAI score ≥7.

The standard PDAI remains an optimal method of diagnosing pouchitis; however, the mPDAI offers similar sensitivity and specificity in diagnosing patients with acute or acute-relapsing pouchitis. This approach simplifies the diagnostic criteria of pouchitis, reduces the cost of diagnosis and avoids delay in determining the histology. In addition, the mPDAI offers better sensitivity and specificity when compared with symptom assessment alone [11].

Pouchitis can be classified in different ways on the basis of symptoms and endoscopic findings. On the basis of disease activity, pouchitis can be divided into remission (regular pouch function with normal frequency of evacuation) or active pouchitis (increased number of bowel movements with endoscopic and histologic features of inflammations consistent with pouchitis) [10].

Active pouchitis can also be divided into mild to moderate (increased stool frequency, urgency and occasional incontinence, usually treated without hospitalization) and severe (which frequently requires hospitalization due to the high number of bowel movement accompanied by incontinence and dehydration) [11–13].

Depending on the symptom duration, it can also be divided into acute, recurrent acute or chronic. Acute pouchitis is a single acute episode resolved following short course of antibiotic treatment. Recurrent acute pouchitis is characterized by recurrent acute episodes, lasting less than 2 weeks, followed by normal pouch function. A symptom duration of more than 4 weeks is the threshold for chronicity [11–13].

Pouchitis can also be classified according to its etiology into idiopathic versus secondary. On the basis of the frequency of clinical episodes, pouchitis can also be divided into: infrequent (1–2 episodes/year), relapsing (more than 3 episodes/year), and continuous or chronic. Finally, pouchitis may also be classified based on the response to antibiotic therapy in antibiotic-responsive, antibiotic-dependent (patients who need continuous antibiotic treatment to maintain remission), and antibiotic-refractory (patients not responding to antibiotics and treated with a wide spread of drugs, from 5-ASA to anti-TNFα) [14].

Chronic antibiotic-refractory pouchitis is one of the leading causes of pouch failure, resulting in permanent diversion or pouch excision [15]. In all cases of chronic refractory pouchitis secondary causes of inflammation should be excluded.

The treatment of pouchitis is largely empirical and is based on different categories of drugs. The first-line therapy for acute pouchitis is represented by antibiotics. The most effective agents are metronidazole and ciprofloxacin. Their use for at least two weeks often results in a rapid response [16].

Metronidazole and ciprofloxacin have been compared in a small randomized trial. Both antibiotics significantly decreased the PDAI score. However, patients treated with ciprofloxacin have a significantly greater benefit as compared with metronidazole in terms of the total PDAI, symptom score, and endoscopic score as well as having fewer adverse events [17]. Budesonide or mesalamine administration with enemas or suppositories is also effective for inducing remission.

Approximately 10–15% of patients with acute pouchitis develop chronic pouchitis, which may be 'treatment responsive' or 'treatment refractory' to a single antibiotic therapy. Patients with antibiotic-dependent pouchitis often require long-term maintenance therapy to keep the disease in remission.

Maintenance agents include probiotics such as VSL#3 and a low dose of antibiotics [18]. The efficacy of probiotics was proven in 2000 with a double-blind study comparing probiotics and placebos for the maintenance of acute relapsing pouchitis after remission which was induced by ciprofloxacin and rifaximin. In this study, only 15% of the patients using probiotics reported a relapse of pouchitis within the 9-month follow-up versus 100% of patients treated with a placebo [19].

In a Cochrane systematic review, VSL#3 was more effective than a placebo in maintaining remission of chronic pouchitis in patients who achieved remission with antibiotics [20]. Proposed mechanisms of probiotics, such as maintenance therapy for pouchitis, include: suppression of resident pathogenic bacteria, stimulation of mucin glycoprotein by intestinal epithelial cells, prevention of adhesion of pathogenic strains to epithelial cells, and induction of host immune responses [21]. The efficacy of probiotics has also been proven in the prevention of pouchitis within the first year after surgery. A randomized, double-blind, placebo-controlled study showed a significantly lower incidence of acute pouchitis in patients treated with VSL#3 when compared with patients treated with a placebo; moreover, patients taking VSL#3 experienced a significant improvement in their quality of life [22].

Patients with chronic, refractory pouchitis do not respond to conventional therapy and often have ongoing symptoms. Combination antibiotic therapy or oral budesonide may be effective [23–25]. The use of biologics in patients with chronic, refractory pouchitis is still under debate. A recent systematic review analyzed their clinical efficacy for the treatment of antibiotic-resistant pouchitis. The data available regarding Infliximab suggest clinical effectiveness in treating antibiotic-refractory or fistulizing pouchitis. The data for adalimumab are much more limited, and sufficient long-term outcomes are lacking [26]. Recent studies have reported the effectiveness of vedolizumab for the treatment of both antibiotic and anti-tumor necrosis alpha refractory pouchitis; however, additional data are required regarding their large-scale use in clinical practice [27, 28].

Surgical management of pouchitis refractory to medical treatment is limited to a defunctioning stoma or pouch excision.

12.3   Pre-pouch Ileitis

An ileal inflammation proximal to the pouch has been described in patients undergoing restorative proctocolectomy for UC, called pre-pouch ileitis. Pre-pouch ileitis usually extends only a short distance beyond the pre-pouch ileal junction and is limited to the distal ileal segment; a pan-small bowel inflammation is uncommon. The incidence of this condition ranges from 3% to 14% in the literature [29, 30].

The pathogenesis of pre-pouch ileitis is still unclear. Some authors have suggested that its presence may indicate CD [31, 32]. For these authors, more than 45% of patients who developed afferent limb ulcers or stenosis had a delayed diagnosis of CD while no ulcers were reported in patients with confirmed UC at follow-up. Conversely, other authors did not find any association between pre-pouch ileitis and CD. McLaughlin et al. described pre-pouch ileitis in 34 out of 742 patients treated with restorative proctocolectomies. None of the patients with pre-pouch ileitis in this study had CD based on histopathological criteria and none were diagnosed with CD during the subsequent follow-up of a median period of more than 12 months [29].

Some studies have reported a close association between pouchitis and pre-pouch ileitis. A study published in 2009 reported pre-pouch ileitis which occurred only in patients with concurrent pouchitis, suggesting that these conditions may have a similar cause [29]. Fecal stasis along with subsequent bacterial overgrowth could be considered the major pathogenesis of both conditions. According to this pathogenesis, both pouchitis and pre-pouch ileitis have similar endoscopic, histological and immunological features.

Association with chronic pouchitis has not been confirmed by subsequent studies. In a study by Bell et al. only half of their patients with pre-pouch ileitis had concomitant pouchitis [33]. It has also been suggested that inflammation of the pouch or pre-pouch ileal loop could be related to distal structuring [34]. A distal stenosis could lead to reflux of the contents of the pouch which could induce ileal inflammation. In the study by Bell, this association was not confirmed; only 20% of the patients with pre-pouch ileitis had significant stenosis of the ileal pouch-anal anastomosis [33].

Some authors have considered pre-pouch ileitis to be the consequence of backwash ileitis. Backwash ileitis is a clinical condition occurring in some patients with UC; it is represented by the extension of the inflammatory process to the terminal portion of the ileum due to reflux of the large bowel contents into the small bowel. Backwash ileitis has been reported in approximately 10% of total colectomy specimens in patients with ulcerative pancolitis; treatment for this condition is the same as for UC uncomplicated by blackwash ileitis. This condition can be asymptomatic or associated with all symptoms of terminal ileitis. The etiology of pre-pouch ileitis may be similar to that of blackwash ileitis. Thus, pre-pouch ileitis may be secondary to reflux of the pouch fecal contents into the pre-pouch ileum. Various studies have identified an association between the presence of backwash ileitis before restorative proctocolectomy and the onset of pre-pouch ileitis at follow-up of patients undergoing IPAA [35].

Contrarily, other studies did not find any association between pre-pouch ileitis and backwash ileitis [29, 36].

An association between pre-pouch ileitis and the chronic use of NSAIDs has been suggested in the literature [37, 38]. The chronic use of NSAIDs could induce injury to the pouch or the pre-pouch ileum, resulting in inflammation, ulcerations and strictures. Non-steroidal anti-inflammatory drug-induced mucosal inflammation does not typically respond to pouchitis-targeted antibiotic therapy and may resolve after the discontinuation of the drugs. However, the long-term use of NSAIDs can cause persistent ulcers or strictures in the small pouch, pouch inlet or outlet, or cuff even after drug withdrawal.

Finally, for some authors pouch design could also influence the onset of pre-pouch ileitis. The pouch configuration may adversely influence vascularization or motility of the neo-terminal ileum conditions which could lead to inflammation of the terminal ileum above the pouch. A higher rate of pre-pouch ileitis has been reported in patients with W pouches rather than in those with J- or S-pouches [33]

Many patients with pre-pouch ileitis can be asymptomatic; more than 20% of patients have no symptoms at the time of diagnosis [29]. In these cases, it can be diagnosed during endoscopies performed for routine follow-up.

Other patients have symptoms related to the ileal inflammation; the main symptoms include increased stool frequency, urgency and bleeding as reported by more than 40% of patients. These disabling symptoms are similar to pouchitis; a differential diagnosis should be considered. Patients with stenosis also report abdominal cramps or obstructive symptoms, such as nausea and vomiting. Subacute obstruction, abdominal flatus or colic, evacuation difficulties and weight loss have been reported by 40%, 33%, 20% and 7% of patients, respectively [33].

More than 50% of patients have poor pouch function; an endoscopic examination of the neo-terminal ileum with biopsies is essential when investigating a patient with non-specific symptoms, including poor function [29].

All patients with clinical suspicion of pre-pouch ileitis should be investigated. A water soluble radiological examination should be performed. (Fig. 12.2)

Varying degrees and combinations of ulcerations, thickening of folds, nodularities, irregularities and strictures are the main radiological findings described. The length of the abnormal bowel varied from 1 to 30 cm. The diagnosis should be confirmed by endoscopic examination. The main endoscopic features include discrete or segmental small and large ulcers, nodularity, exudate and/or inflammatory pseudopolyps in the afferent limb of the pouch (Fig. 12.3).

Inflammation of the ileal segment above the pouch can be associated with strictures of the ileum. All patients with symptomatic stenosis should be evaluated with magnetic resonance or computed tomography enterography

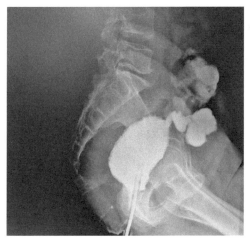

Fig. 12.2 Pre-pouch ileitis with stenosis at the inlet of the pouch

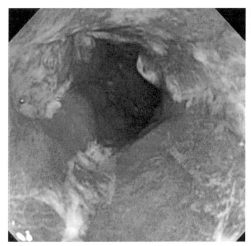

Fig. 12.3 Endoscopic finding of pre-pouch ileitis

in order to define the length of the intestinal stenosis and the presence of extraintestinal complications, such as abscesses or fistulas. These radiological examinations are very important after the failure of medical therapy in patients who should undergo surgical procedures (Fig. 12.4).

Patients with pre-pouch ileitis can be treated using different approaches. Patients without symptoms should be followed with periodic endoscopies without any specific medical treatment; spontaneous remissions have been described. In symptomatic cases, medical treatment should be used. Patients without stenosis should be treated with antibiotics, such as ciprofloxacin alone or in combination with metronidazole. The combination of these antibiotics used for at least 4 weeks is effective; in selected patients, symptomatic remission

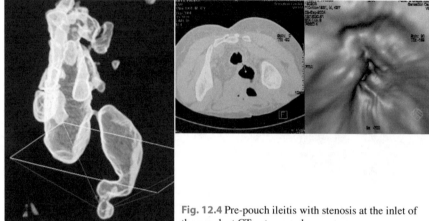

Fig. 12.4 Pre-pouch ileitis with stenosis at the inlet of the pouch at CT enterography

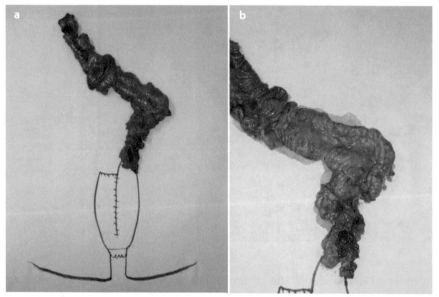

Fig. 12.5 Resection of the stenotic ileum above the pouch

associated with resolution of the pre-pouch ileitis or a reduction in the length of distal ileum involved has been reported in more than 80% of cases [29].

In cases of persistent inflammation after antibiotic therapy, patients should be treated with 5-ASA or budesonide orally. In patients resistant to previous medical approaches, the administration of infliximab can be attempted. Infliximab has also been shown to be effective in the treatment of extensive pre-

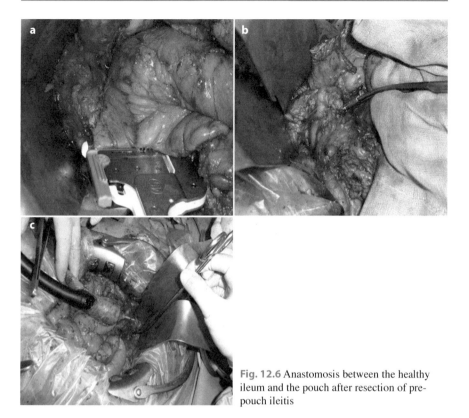

Fig. 12.6 Anastomosis between the healthy ileum and the pouch after resection of pre-pouch ileitis

pouch ileitis. Various studies have reported the efficacy of biologics in inducing the clinical and endoscopic remission of ileal inflammation [29, 35].

In selected patients with a short pre-pouch stenosis, endoscopic dilatation can be attempted. This procedure should be performed only on patients with a single stenosis, shorter than 3 cm. The dilatation should be maintained with further periodic endoscopic dilatations.

After failure of medical or endoscopic treatments symptomatic patients require surgical intervention. The main surgical treatment of this condition is resection of the proximal ileal loop above the pouch (Fig. 12.5).

Subsequently, a new anastomosis between the healthy ileum and the pouch must be fashioned (Fig. 12.6).

In the majority of cases, this anastomosis is obtained with a diverting ileostomy. In all patients undergoing ileal resection for pre-pouch ileitis, it is important to preserve the vascularization of the pouch itself. According to this, dissection of the ileal mesentery should be performed close to intestinal wall.

Selected cases with a short stenosis of the inlet of the pouch should be surgically treated without resection of the ileum. A Heineke-Mikulicz strictureplasty can be attempted to treat the stenosis; in this case, a diverting ileostomy should be fashioned.

During their lifetime, some patients may require sequential resections for relapse; this condition can lead to pouch failure. In this case, an end ileostomy with or without removal of the pouch must be performed.

12.4 Cuffitis

Currently, a double-stapled anastomosis is the preferred technique used for fashioning an ileoanal anastomosis. This procedure is simpler to perform and less likely to result in functional and septic complications. During a stapled restorative proctocolectomy, a 1.5–2 cm cuff of diseased columnar epithelium remains at the location proximal to the anal transitional zone. This area, called the "columnar cuff" or "rectal cuff," is at risk for developing symptomatic inflammation. Cuffitis was defined as inflammation of the rectal cuff in the area between the anastomosis and the dentate line on endoscopy and histology, with or without minimal inflammation of the pouch body (Fig. 12.7) [39].

The etiology and pathogenesis of cuffitis are not clear. Cuffitis has been considered a variant form of UC in the rectal cuff. The risk factors for cuffitis onset are preoperative toxic megacolon or fulminant colitis, the preoperative use of biologics and stapled anastomosis without mucosectomy [40]. However, cuffitis can also occur in patients who had a hand-sewn anastomosis with mucosectomy since it is difficult to ensure a complete mucosectomy, and some patients will have islands of residual rectal mucosa [41].

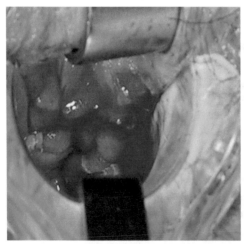

Fig. 12.7 Cuffitis

Cuffitis could be considered a residual form of UC with a similar clinical presentation. The clinical course is the same as active colitis with attenuated symptoms; some authors have defined cuffitis as a "little ulcerative colitis". The main symptoms are increased bowel movements, urgency, bleeding and perianal pain and 2–15% of patients are symptomatic [39, 40]. Cuffitis can cause pouch dysfunction with symptoms similar to those of pouchitis, CD of the pouch or irritable pouch syndrome.

Diagnosis can be reached by endoscopy, but care has to be taken to examine the cuff of the columnar epithelium between the dentate line and pouch-anal anastomosis. Endoscopic features are the same as those of UC; the main findings are friability, nodularity and ulcerations [39].

The first-line therapy for cuffitis is topical mesalamine and/or topical corticosteroid agents. In an open-label trial, 14 consecutive patients with cuffitis treated with 5-ASA suppositories twice daily experienced a reduction in the inflammation of the rectal cuff at endoscopy and histology with a reduction in bloody bowel movements and extraintestinal manifestations [42]. The association of topical 5-ASA with corticosteroid therapy appears to be effective in 50–70% of the patients treated [40, 42]. Systemic agents are rarely needed. The use of local injections of biologics has recently also been reported for the treatment of cuffitis with good clinical effects.

Refractory cuffitis remains a therapeutic challenge. Patients with refractory cuffitis should be evaluated for other disease processes at or around the cuff, such as fistula and chronic anastomotic leaks. Refractory cuffitis can also be a sign of CD of the pouch or it could be due to chronic ischemia; in fact, ischemic features on endoscopy and histology have been found in some patients with refractory cuffitis, suggesting a contribution of this factor to its development [42].

Wu et al. reported cases of resolution of refractory cuffitis after ileostomy and lysis of adhesion surgery. The mechanism with which cuffitis had a favorable response to lysis of adhesion surgery with temporary diversion ileostomy was not clear. This supports the notion that cuffitis may have different etiopathogenetic pathways, ranging from an inflammatory bowel disease-like inflammatory process to an ischemic entity. The therapeutic effect of lysis of adhesion surgery may contribute to the promotion of blood flow [43]. Refractory cuffitis may benefit from endoscopic injection of long-acting corticosteroids.

Untreated or unhealed cuffitis can evolve with the onset of deep ulcerations of the anal canal and development of fistulas such as pouch-anal or pouch-vaginal fistulas; this condition may lead to pouch failure.

Finally, dysplasia and cancer have been reported in the rectal cuff. In a review of 23 reports, with a total of 2040 patients who had undergone IPAA for UC, the pooled risk of dysplasia was 1.13% in the rectal cuff [44].

Pouch failure due to cuffitis is approximately 13.3% [40]. The causes of pouch failure can be refractory cuffitis, CD of the cuff, chronic ischemia or concurrent surgical complications, such as fistulizing disease.

Patients with pouch failure due to refractory cuffitis can be treated with permanent diversion with pouch excision, permanent diversion without pouch excision or redo-surgery. In these cases, redo-surgery includes both redo-pouch and redo-anastomosis. A redo-pouch is suggested in patients with cuffitis and concomitant surgical complications such as pouch-anal or pouch-vaginal fistulas. Patients with only refractory cuffitis could be treated with redo-anastomosis. Patients treated with redo-surgery require a hand-sewn anastomosis with mucosectomy.

12.5   Anastomotic Stenosis

Anastomotic stricture is a frequent condition which has been reported in 5–15% of patients with IPAA [13, 15].

The anal canal typically narrows to some extent after IPAA. A lumen of 1–2 cm in diameter is considered satisfactory. An anastomotic stricture can be defined as a symptomatic narrowing of the ileoanal anastomosis requiring either two or more outpatient dilatations or at least one dilatation under anesthesia.

Strictures can occur in both stapled and hand-sewn anastomoses [15]. Strictures can be fibrotic or inflammatory (non-fibrotic) in nature. Based on the cause, strictures can be related to inappropriate surgical techniques, ischemia, concurrent use of NSAIDs or CD. The fibrosis can be due to partial dehiscence of the IPAA or marginal anastomotic ischemia. The main reason for chronic ischemia is high tension in the mesentery. High tension in the mesentery is due to bad lengthening of the ileum performed before fashioning of the ileo-anal anastomosis; this condition is associated with an increased risk of postoperative complications, such as early anastomotic leaks or long term anastomotic stenosis with a high rate of pouch failure [45].

An anastomotic stricture could be asymptomatic at the beginning. If severe, the stricture may obstruct the outlet of the pouch and result in evacuation problems, pouch dilatation and bacterial overgrowth. The main symptoms are the increased number of bowel movements, bowel fragmentation and incontinence due to the exclusive passage of liquid stool.

Stenosis can be differentiated into short and soft, or long and fibrotic. A short and soft stenosis is frequently related to residual inflammation or to the natural narrowing of the anastomosis over time. This type of stricture can easily be treated with mechanical dilatations using Hegar's dilators (nos. 13 to 18). Hegar's dilators can be used to gradually dilate mild strictures. Severe stricture needs a first dilatation under general anesthesia in a day surgery operating room. Subsequently the dilatation should be maintained with self-dilatations using Hegar's dilators. The overall success of self-mechanical dilatation is approximately 75% in treated patients [46]. Inflammatory stenosis could benefit from concomitant treatment with 5-ASA medication or local steroids. Local injections of steroids have also been successfully reported in the literature [47].

Long and fibrotic stenosis are associated with septic postoperative complications or chronic ischemia. These strictures do not respond to mechanical dilatations and required redo-surgery, which is not always possible. Fibrotic stenosis is associated with a higher risk of pouch failure.

12.6   Crohn Disease of the Pouch

Crohn's disease of the pouch can be identified in three different scenarios. It can occur after IPAA, which is performed intentionally in some patients having Crohn's colitis with no previous small intestinal or perianal disease. A first series of IPAAs in 31 highly selected patients with Crohn's colitis without ileal or perianal involvement was reported by Panis et al. in 1996 [48]. There were no significant differences between patients with CD and UC according to early postoperative complications and long-term functional results with a 5-year pouch failure of 6.5%.

Crohn's disease can also be found inadvertently in the colectomy specimens of patients with a preoperative diagnosis of UC (incidental diagnosis) or, finally, it can develop de novo in patients having a preoperative diagnosis of UC and without evidence of CD on the surgical specimen (delayed diagnosis).

The cumulative frequencies of CD of the pouch range from 2.7% to 13% [49–51]. Clinically, CD of the pouch can be classified into inflammatory, fibrostenotic or fistulizing phenotypes; these phenotypes may not be static. For example, inflammatory CD can progress into fibrostenotic or fistulizing disease. Moreover, CD may not be limited to the pouch, and its manifestations can occur in any part of the gastrointestinal tract. There are various clinical features, and the clinical manifestation could be similar to other conditions, such as pouchitis, pre-pouch ileitis and fistulizing disease.

The diagnosis of CD of the pouch should be based on a combined assessment of symptoms, endoscopy, histology and radiography.

The main endoscopic features of CD of the pouch include the presence of afferent limb ulcers and/or strictures in the setting of ulcerated strictures of the pouch inlet, and the presence of ulcers or stricture in other parts of the small bowel. Typically, CD ileitis is characterized by discrete ulcers in the distal neoterminal ileum (10 cm beyond the pouch inlet) and ulcerated stricture at the pouch inlet. In contrast, backwash ileitis from diffuse pouchitis is characterized by the presence of continuous endoscopic and histologic inflammation from the pouch to the distal neoterminal ileum (typically within 10 cm of the pouch inlet) with a widely patent pouch inlet.

It also is important to differentiate CD from surgery-associated stricture fistulizing complications. This distinction can be difficult to make. In clinical practice, CD of the pouch should be suspected if a patient develops de novo fistulas more than 6 to 12 months after ileostomy take-down in the absence of postoperative leak, abscess and sepsis. CD should also be investigated in patients with refractory cuffitis.

Treatment of CD of the pouch is difficult, and requires a combined approach of medical therapy, endoscopic treatment and surgical procedures. Fistulizing CD of the pouch is associated with a high risk of pouch failure [52].

Crohn's disease of the pouch can also negatively influence functional outcomes and quality of life in patients undergoing restorative proctocolectomy. Similar results obtained in UC have been reported only in selected patients intentionally undergoing IPAA with a preoperative diagnosis of CD [48]. A recent Cleveland Clinic study compared functional outcomes and quality of life in patients undergoing IPAA with an intentional, incidental or delayed diagnosis of CD. The data obtained reported a higher pouch retention rate in patients intentionally or incidentally treated with IPAA when compared with patients having a delayed diagnosis of CD. Patients with a delayed diagnosis of CD have higher rates of pouch-anal and pouch-vaginal fistulas, chronic pouchitis and anastomotic strictures with a subsequently higher rate of pouch failure. Moreover, patients with an intentional or incidental diagnosis of CD reported better scores in functional outcome evaluation [53].

12.7   Irritable Pouch Syndrome

Irritable pouch syndrome is a new functional disorder in patients undergoing restorative proctocolectomy described for the first time by Shen et al. in 2002 [54]. Patients with irritable pouch syndrome reported significantly lower health-related quality-of-life scores than patients with healthy pouches [55].

The pathogenesis of this condition is still unclear. It can be attributed to psychosocial factors [55], visceral hypersensitivity [56] and enterochromaffin cell hyperplasia of the pouch mucosa [57]. Currently, the diagnosis of irritable pouch syndrome is based on the exclusion of organic complications of the pouch in patients with increased frequency of bowel movements with a change in stool consistency, abdominal pain, and perianal or pelvic discomfort. The absence of endoscopic and histologic inflammation has been reported in all cases of irritable pouch syndrome. The clinical features of this disease are similar to those of pouchitis and other disorders of the pouch, and to those of irritable bowel syndrome. In patients with a supposed diagnosis of irritable pouch syndrome, inflammatory and/or surgical complications of the pouch must be excluded. Moreover, celiac disease, lactose or fructose intolerance, and proximal small-bowel bacterial overgrowth should also be investigated. Treatment of irritable pouch syndrome is empiric, and therapeutic agents include antidiarrheals, antispasmodics and tricyclic antidepressants.

12.8   Mega Pouch

A mega pouch is an unusual condition represented by an abnormal enlargement of the body of the pouch which could lead to functional dysfunction. Different causes can be associated with this condition. Initially, many surgeons believed that pouches with a wide volume could represent a better reservoir for ileal stool and pouches of more than 20 cm in length were proposed. This initial conviction has not been confirmed by functional studies. A too large reservoir resulted in poorer functional outcomes due to the incomplete emptying associated with bowel movement fragmentation. A mega pouch could be the consequence of the torsion of pouch on its axis or associated with severe strictures of the pouch-anal anastomosis with subsequent difficulties in emptying.

Patients with mega pouch often report clinical dysfunctions which worsen over time. The initial symptoms are mainly associated with incomplete evacuations with increased bowel movements, increased liquid stools and tenesmus. Subsequently, patients could present severe difficulties with evacuation requiring the periodic use of enemas or pouch intubation due to reduction of the contractility of the pouch. A diagnosis can be reached using endoscopy or radiological pouchography with water soluble contrast.

Symptomatic patients can be treated with the periodic use of enemas or pouch intubations; however, the resolution of pouch enlargement can be obtained only with surgical intervention.

Surgical therapy includes both redo-pouch and pouchplasty, which can result in symptomatic resolution and maintenance of satisfactory function. Redo-pouches require the removal of the mega-pouch followed, when possible, by the fashioning of a new pouch using a hand-sewn anastomosis. Pouchplasty is a complex procedure performed for reducing the volume of a huge pouch; during the procedure, the vascularization of the ileum must be carefully preserved (Fig. 12.8).

For preventing the onset of mega pouch, the pouch dimension should be tailored to the body size of the patient.

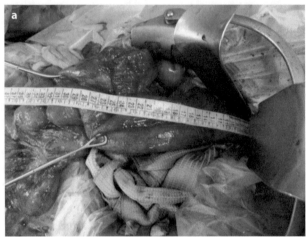

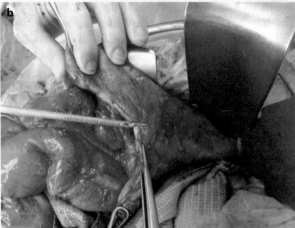

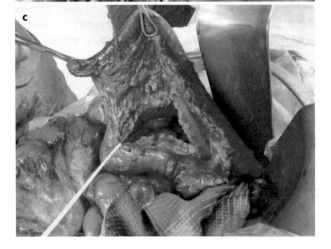

Fig. 12.8 Pouchplasty. **a** Evaluation of the size of the mega pouch. **b** Resection of the upper part of the mega pouch preserving distal ileal vascularization. **c** Preservation of vascularization of the distal part of the pouch. **d** Resection of the distal part of the mega pouch using linear stapler. **e** Section of the pre-pouch ileum using linear stapler. **f** Double stapled anastomosis between the pre-pouch ileum and the resized pouch

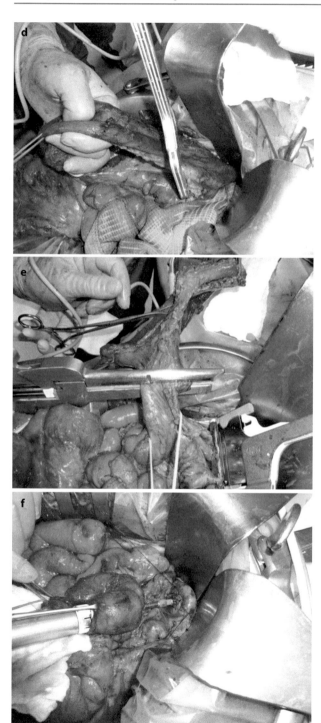

References

1. Hurst RD, Molinari M, Chung TP et al (1996) Prospective study of the incidence, timing and treatment of pouchitis in 104 consecutive patients after restorative proctocolectomy. Arch Surg 131(5):497–500
2. Meagher AP, Farouk R, Dozois RR et al (1998) J ileal pouch-anal anastomosis for chronic ulcerative colitis: complications and long-term outcome in 1310 patients. Br J Surg 85(6):800–803
3. Penna C, Dozois R, Tremaine W et al (1996) Pouchitis after ileal pouch-anal anastomosis for ulcerative colitis occurs with increased frequency in patients with associated primary sclerosing cholangitis. Gut 38(2):234–239
4. Landy J, Al-Hassi HO, McLaughlin SD et al (2012) Etiology of pouchitis. Inflamm Bowel Dis 18(6):1146–1155
5. Carter MJ, Di Giovine FS, Cox A et al (2001) The interleukin 1 receptor antagonist gene allele 2 as a predictor of pouchitis following colectomy and IPAA in ulcerative colitis. Gastroenterology 121(4):805–811
6. Meier CB, Hegazi RA, Aisenberg J et al (2005) Innate immune receptor genetic polymorphisms in pouchitis: is CARD15 susceptibility factor? Inflamm Bowel Dis 11(11):965–971
7. Achkar JP, Al-Haddad M, Lashner B et al (2005) Differentiating risk factors for acute and chronic pouchitis. Clin Gastroenterol Hepatol 3(1):60–66
8. Fleshner P, Ippoliti A, Dubinsky M et al (2007) A prospective multivariate analysis of clinical factors associated with pouchitis after ileal pouch-anal anastomosis. Clin Gastroenterol Hepatol 5(8):952–958
9. Sandborn WJ, Tremaine WJ, Batts KP et al (1994) Pouchitis after ileal pouch-anal anastomosis: a Pouchitis Disease Activity Index. Mayo Clin Proc 69(5):409–415
10. Shen B, Achkar J-P, Lashner BA et al (2001) Endoscopic and histologic evaluation together with symptom assessment are required to diagnose pouchitis. Gastroenterology 121(2):261–267
11. Shen B, Achkar JP, Connor JT et al (2003) Modified pouchitis disease activity index: a simplified approach to the diagnosis of pouchitis. Dis Colon Rectum 46(6):748–753
12. Sandborn WJ (1996) Pouchitis: risk factors, frequency, natural history, classification and public health prospective. In: McLeod RS, Martin F, Sutherland LR et al (eds) Trends in inflammatory bowel disease therapy. Kluwer Academic Publishers, Dordrecht
13. Shen B, Remzi FH, Lavery IC et al (2008) A proposed classification of ileal pouch disorders and associated complications after restorative proctocolectomy. Clin Gastroenterol Hepatol 6(2):145–158
14. Pardi DS, D'Haens G, Shen B et al (2009) Clinical guidelines for the management of pouchitis. Inflamm Bowel Dis 15(9):1424–1431
15. Fazio VW, Kiran RP, Remzi FH et al (2013) Ileal pouch anal anastomosis: analysis of outcome and quality of life in 3707 patients. Ann Surg 257(4):679–685
16. Sandborn W, McLeod R, Jewell D (2000) Pharmacotherapy for inducing and maintaining remission in pouchitis. Cochrane Database Syst Rev 2000(2):CD001176
17. Shen B, Achkar JP, Lashner BA et al (2001) A randomized clinical trial of ciprofloxacin and metronidazole to treat acute pouchitis. Inflamm Bowel Dis 7(4):301–305
18. Mimura T, Rizzello F, Helwig U et al (2004) Once daily high dose probiotic therapy (VSL#3) for maintaining remission in recurrent or refractory pouchitis. Gut 53(1):108–114
19. Gionchetti P, Rizzello F, Venturi A et al (2000) Oral bacteriotherapy as maintenance treatment in patients with chronic pouchitis: a double-blind, placebo-controlled trial. Gastroenterology 119(2):305–309
20. Singh S, Stroud AM, Holubar SD et al (2015) Treatment and prevention of pouchitis after ileal pouch-anal anastomosis for chronic ulcerative colitis. Cochrane Database Syst Rev 2015(11):CD001176

21. Sartor RB (2000) Probiotics in chronic pouchitis: restoring luminal microbial balance. Gastroenterology 119(2):584–587
22. Gionchetti P, Rizzello F, Helwig U et al (2003) Prophylaxis of pouchitis onset with probiotic therapy: a double-blind, placebo-controlled trial. Gastroenterology 124(5):1202–1209
23. Gionchetti P, Rizzello F, Poggioli G et al (2007) Oral budesonide in the treatment of chronic refractory pouchitis. Aliment Pharmacol Ther 25(10):1231–1236
24. Gionchetti P, Rizzello F, Venturi A et al (1999) Antibiotic combination therapy in patients with chronic, treatment-resistant pouchitis. Aliment Pharmacol Ther 13(6):713–718
25. Mimura T, Rizzello F, Helwig U et al (2002) Four-week open-label trial of metronidazole and ciprofloxacin for the treatment of recurrent or refractory pouchitis. Aliment Pharmacol Ther 16(5):909–917
26. Herfarth HH, Long MD, Isaacs KL (2015) Use of biologics in pouchitis: a systematic review. J Clin Gastroenterol 49(8):647–654
27. Mir F, Yousef MH, Partyka EK, Tahan V (2017) Successful treatment of chronic refractory pouchitis with vedolizumab. Int J Colorectal Dis 32(10):1517–1518
28. Philpott J, Ashburn J, Shen B (2017) Efficacy of vedolizumab in patients with antibiotic and anti-tumor necrosis alpha refractory pouchitis. Inflamm Bowel Dis 23(1):E5–E6
29. McLaughlin SD, Clark SK, Bell AJ et al (2009) Incidence and short-term implications of prepouch ileitis following restorative proctocolectomy with ileal pouch-anal anastomosis for ulcerative colitis. Dis Colon Rectum 52(5):879–883
30. Kuisma J, Jarvinen H, Kahri A, Färkkilä M (2004) Factors associated with disease activity of pouchitis after surgery for ulcerative colitis. Scand J Gastroenterol 39(6):544–548
31. Wolf JM, Achkar JP, Lashner BA et al (2004) Afferent limb ulcers predict Crohn's disease in patients with ileal pouch-anal anastomosis. Gastroenterology 126(7):1686–1691
32. Pardi DS, Sandborn WJ (2006) Systematic review: the management of pouchitis. Aliment Pharmacol Ther 23(8):1087–1096
33. Bell AJ, Price AB, Forbes A et al (2006) Pre-pouch ileitis: a disease of the ileum in ulcerative colitis after restorative proctocolectomy. Colorectal Dis 8(5):402–410
34. Scott AD, Phillips RK (1989) Ileitis and pouchitis after colectomy for ulcerative colitis. Br J Surg 76(7): 668–669
35. McLaughlin SD, Clark SK, Bell AJ et al (2009) An open study of antibiotics for the treatment of pre-pouch ileitis following restorative proctocolectomy with ileal pouch-anal anastomosis. Aliment Pharmacol Ther 29(1):69–74
36. Schmidt CM, Lazenby AJ, Hendrickson RJ, Sitzmann JV (1998) Preoperative terminal ileal and colonic resection histopathology predicts risk of pouchitis in patients after ileoanal pull-through procedure. Ann Surg 227(5): 654–662; discussion 663–665
37. Iwata T, Yamamoto T, Umegae S, Matsumoto K (2007) Pouchitis and pre-pouch ileitis developed after restorative proctocolectomy for ulcerative colitis: a case report. World J Gastroenterol 13(4):643–646
38. Slatter C, Girgis S, Huynh H, El-Matary W (2008) Pre-pouch ileitis after colectomy in paediatric ulcerative colitis. Acta Paediatr 97(3):381–383
39. Thompson-Fawcett MW, Mortensen NJ, Warren BF (1999) "Cuffitis" and inflammatory changes in the columnar cuff, anal transitional zone, and ileal reservoir after stapled pouch-anal anastomosis. Dis Colon Rectum 42(3):348–355
40. Wu B, Lian L, Li Y et al (2013) Clinical course of cuffitis in ulcerative colitis patients with restorative proctocolectomy and ileal pouch-anal anastomoses. Inflamm Bowel Dis 19(2):404–410
41. O'Connell PR, Pemberton JH, Weiland LH et al (1987) Does rectal mucosa regenerate after ileoanal anastomosis? Dis Colon Rectum 30(1):1–5
42. Shen B, Lashner BA, Bennett AE et al (2004) Treatment of rectal cuff inflammation (cuffitis) in patients with ulcerative colitis following restorative proctocolectomy and ileal pouch-anal anastomosis. Am J Gastroenterol 99(8):1527–1531
43. Wu B, Liu X, Shen B (2013) Refractory cuffitis resolved after temporary ileostomy and lysis of adhesion surgery. Inflamm Bowel Dis 19(3):E32–33

44. Scarpa M, van Koperen PJ, Ubbink DT et al (2007) Systematic review of dysplasia after restorative proctocolectomy for ulcerative colitis. Br J Surg 94(5):534–545
45. Wu XR, Kirat HT, Xhaja X et al (2014) The impact of mesenteric tension on pouch outcome and quality of life in patients undergoing restorative proctocolectomy. Colorectal Dis 16(12):986–994
46. Gentilini L, Coscia M, Lombardi PM et al (2016) Ileal pouch-anal anastomosis 20 years later: is it still a good surgical option for patients with ulcerative colitis? Int J Colorectal Dis 31(12):1835–1843
47. Lucha PA Jr, Fticsar JE, Francis MJ (2005) The strictured anastomosis: successful treatment by corticosteroid injections-report of three cases and review of the literature. Dis Colon Rectum 48(4): 862–865
48. Panis Y, Poupard B, Nemeth J et al (1996) Ileal pouch/anal anastomosis for Crohn's disease. Lancet 347(9005):854–857
49. Keighley MR (2000) The final diagnosis in pouch patients for presumed ulcerative colitis may change to Crohn's disease: patients should be warned of the consequences. Acta Chir Iugosl 47(4 Suppl 1):27–31
50. Peyrègne V, Francois Y, Gilly F-N et al (2000) Outcome of ileal pouch after secondary diagnosis of Crohn's disease. Int J Colorectal Dis 15(1):49–53
51. Goldstein NS, Sanford WW, Bodzin JH (1997) Crohn's-like complications in patients with ulcerative colitis after total proctocolectomy and ileal pouch-anal anastomosis. Am J Surg Pathol 21(11):1343–1353
52. Shen B, Fazio VW, Remzi FH et al (2007) Clinical features and quality of life in patients with different phenotypes of Crohn's disease of the ileal pouch. Dis Colon Rectum 50(9):1450–1459
53. Melton GB, Fazio VW, Kiran RP et al (2008) Long-term outcomes with ileal pouch-anal anastomosis and Crohn's disease: pouch retention and implications of delayed diagnosis. Ann Surg 248(4):608–616
54. Shen B, Achkar J-P, Lashner BA et al (2002) Irritable pouch syndrome: a new category of diagnosis for symptomatic patients with ileal pouch-anal anastomosis. Am J Gastroenterol 97(4):972–977
55. Shen B, Fazio VW, Remzi FH et al (2005) Comprehensive evaluation of inflammatory and noninflammatory sequelae of ileal pouch-anal anastomoses. Am J Gastroenterol 100(1):93–101
56. Shen B, Sanmiguel C, Parsi M et al (2004) Irritable pouch syndrome (IPS) is characterized by visceral hypersensitivity and poor quality-of-life (QOL) score. Gastroenterology 126(Suppl 2):A124
57. Shen B, Liu W, Remzi FH et al (2008) Enterochromaffin cell hyperplasia in irritable pouch syndrome. Am J Gastroenterol 103(9):2293–2300

Management and Treatment of Fistulas after Surgical Treatment of Ulcerative Colitis

13

Gilberto Poggioli, Laura Vittori, and Silvio Laureti

13.1   Introduction

Ileal-pouch fistulas after total proctocolectomy and pouch-anal anastomosis are a rare and overwhelming complication for patients and a challenging problem for surgeons. In patients with ileal pouch-anal anastomosis (IPAA), fistulous tracts can originate at any level of the pouch and anal canal, and they can extend into any adjacent hollow organs or to the skin.

Even though several studies have assessed pouch-vaginal fistula formation, little has been published regarding overall perianal fistula formation after restorative proctocolectomy. Pouch-anal or pouch-vaginal fistulas may occur at any time following restorative proctocolectomy, with an incidence of 2.6–14%, depending on the length of the follow-up [1–3]. A fistula after ileoanal pouch construction may occur in the form of a leak in the early period, but it is more frequently seen as a late complication some months after the procedure. In the majority of cases, the ileoanal anastomosis is the origin of early fistulas presenting with pelvic and perianal sepsis, and most likely associated with the technical aspects of the operation.

Several factors have been associated with the development of early pouch fistulas, including preoperative colorectal pathology and medical therapy, operative technique, and postoperative pelvic sepsis. There are controversial reports as to whether the type of anastomosis in IPAA predisposes to the development of pouch fistulas. A prospective randomized trial comparing hand-sewn and stapled anastomoses found no differences over a follow-up period of 15–27 years [4–7]. In fact, more than the incidence, the type of anastomosis

S. Laureti (✉)
Department of Medical and Surgical Sciences, University of Bologna, S. Orsola-Malpighi Hospital
Bologna, Italy
e-mail: silvio.laureti2@unibo.it

G. Poggioli (Ed), *Ulcerative Colitis,*
Updates in Surgery
DOI: 10.1007/978-88-470-3977-3_13, © Springer-Verlag Italia 2019

performed (hand-sewn vs. stapled) influences the therapeutic approach of early post-surgical fistulas. In hand-sewn anastomoses, in cases of a fistula arising in the immediate postoperative period (within 3–4 days after surgery), re-suturing is the treatment of choice; in the case of delayed dehiscence (more than 5–6 days), immediate intervention is important to drain the pelvic sepsis, due to the risk of pouch failure.

By contrast, late fistulas (defined as occurring more than 6 months after ileostomy takedown), usually present as an abscess, or with drainage and pain. These fistulas tend to originate above or, more frequently, distal to the ileoanal anastomosis and result from a more diverse range of causes. A delayed diagnosis of Crohn's disease (CD) is the most common etiology reported. In fact, there is a subset of IPAA patients who undergo restorative proctocolectomy for presumed mucosal ulcerative colitis (UC) or indeterminate colitis (IC) who subsequently develop CD-like complications. Such CD-like complications include fistulous disease involving the perineum in 30–60% of patients and subsequent pouch failure in 30–50% of cases [8–10]. Patient age has also been investigated as a marker for increased complications after restorative proctocolectomy. No significant differences have been noted in complications or functional outcomes in either the elderly or the pediatric population [11].

The classification of pouch-anal fistulas is important to ensure that the correct therapy, either surgical and/or medical, is chosen. Furthermore, appropriate classification is clinically important, given that patients with simple fistulous tracts have better outcomes [12]. Simple fistulas are characterized as submucosal or low inter-sphincteric with only one opening, and they are neither associated with an abscess nor connected to an adjacent structure [13]. However, the occurrence of simple fistulas is a rare event after IPAA. Complex fistulas are much more frequent and involve a significant portion of the anal sphincter (i.e., high trans-sphincteric, supra- or extra-sphincteric), are pouch-vaginal, have multiple openings, "horseshoes" and are usually associated with perianal abscess and/or connect to an adjacent structure [13]. Most commonly, a fistula takes the form of a pouch–vaginal fistula. In females, pouch-vaginal fistulas occur in 2–17% of patients [14], most often at the pouch-anal anastomosis (77%), followed by the body of the pouch (13%), and below the anastomosis. After the ileal pouch has been fashioned, the incidence of fistulas increases overtime. While the majority present in the first year after surgery and a quarter before closure of the ileostomy [5, 15], an increasing number are presenting more than 10 years after the fashioning of the ileal pouch. The incidence of pouch-vaginal fistulas relates to a number of factors including a late diagnosis of Crohn's disease, peri-pouch sepsis and technical factors. Pouch-vaginal fistulas remain an ever-present concern in females undergoing IPAA since they cause major morbidity and have a high rate of pouch failure (22–35%) [16, 17].

Several operative techniques have been described to control perianal sepsis and, ultimately, heal the fistulous tract; however, due to the individual complexity of the fistulas, optimal management continues to be controversial. In patients with pouch-anal and pouch-vaginal fistulas, pouch failure, defined as a definitive ileostomy with or without pouch excision, remains high and is reported in 21–30% of patients with fistulas [18, 19]; however, the factors contributing to pouch excision remain poorly defined.

13.2   Diagnosis

Diagnosis is a crucial aspect in the management of fistulizing complications of IPAA inasmuch as the findings influence the therapeutic strategy. Based on the data in the literature related to the diagnostic algorithm for complex perianal fistulas in CD, various tools have been described, including examination under anesthetic (EUA), fistulography and imaging by endoscopic ultrasonography or magnetic resonance (MRI).

As the presence of concomitant mucosal inflammation has prognostic and therapeutic relevance, endoscopic examination of the pouch should be carried out routinely in the initial evaluation. Fistulas may be seen at fluoroscopy after an infusion of water-soluble contrast material into the pouch. However, pouchography has low sensitivity for the detection of narrow fistulas, possibly because transrectal contrast material often follows the path of the bowel lumen rather than opacifying the fistula. Similarly, computed tomography may not always depict fistulas; sensitivity is reported to be as low as 33%. Pelvic MRI should be the initial procedure together with EUA because it is accurate and non-invasive, although it is not needed routinely in simple fistulas [20]. Anorectal ultrasound requires expertise, but it can be equivalent to MRI in complementing EUA if anastomotic stenosis has been excluded. Fistulography is not recommended since it does not add any data regarding the relationship between the fistulous tract and the sphincters.

Examination under anesthesia is considered to be the gold standard only in the hands of an experienced surgeon since it is reported to be the most sensitive examination, with an accuracy of 90% [21]. It has the advantage of permitting concomitant surgery. MRI has an accuracy of 76–100% as compared with EUA for fistulas and may provide additional information. Anorectal ultrasound has an accuracy of 56–100%, especially when performed by experts in conjunction with hydrogen peroxide enhancement. Any of these methods can be combined with endoscopy to assess the presence or absence of perianastomotic inflammation in the body of the pouch; the presence of histologic evidence of granulomas or pyloric gland metaplasia would also suggest a diagnosis of CD [22].

Combination of instrumental and clinical evaluation with a high level of accuracy is recommended when assessing the results of treatments, both medical and surgical, since clinical evaluation alone, such as the "absence of drainage following gentle finger pressure on the external fistula orifice", is not always consistent with real healing of the fistulous tracts [23].

13.3   Treatment

13.3.1   Early Pouch-anal Fistulas

The presentation of pouch-anal fistulas varies according to the time of occurrence and etiology. A fistula at the anastomotic level is usually the later presentation of an initial anastomotic leak, and it can track to various adjacent locations, such as the prostate, urethra, vagina, gluteal muscle space or skin. The main risk factors for septic complication after IPAA are represented by long-term steroid and immunosuppressive therapies (mainly biologics) and malnutrition. The fashioning of a diverting temporary ileostomy can reduce the risk of this type of complication.

The choice of treatment for postoperative fistula is conditioned by the subsequent clinical picture (Fig. 13.1). In fact, in the case of small, completely asymptomatic "radiological fistula", conservative treatment is usually effective. Subsequent development of a chronic perianastomotic sinus can be treated endoscopically or surgically by the unroofing technique [24]. On the other hand, in cases of clinically relevant fistulas, an abdominoperineal surgical combined approach with fecal diversion and drainage of the pelvic sepsis is mandatory, eventually resulting in healing of the fistulous tract by second intention. Anastomotic fistulas often cause pelvic sepsis, an important postoperative complication of IPAA, described in the literature in percentages ranging from 5% to 24% of patients [25] and representing the main surgical cause of pouch failure. It should be pointed out, however, that fistulas could be the consequence of pelvic sepsis (e.g., due to infection of a pelvic hematoma). The risk of pouch failure with definitive ileostomy has now been reduced (from 5.8 to 1.1%) in high volume referral centers, but treatment of septic complications, usually by means of a redo pouch or a redo anastomosis, is still technically demanding [26]. Redo procedures allow salvage of the pouch-anal anastomosis in up to 80% of patients in specialized centers, although the functional results could be considerably worse than unsuccessful primary procedures.

Finally, recent preliminary reports show encouraging outcomes after vacuum-assisted closure therapy as the unique treatment for anastomotic leaks following IPAA without any additional surgery [27]. Endo-Sponge (B. Braun Medical B.V., Melsungen, Germany) is an open-pored polyurethane sponge specifically designed for small leaks; it is connected to a vacuum suction bottle which is placed endoscopically in the presacral cavity in order to create a constant negative pressure, allowing progressive reduction in the size of the

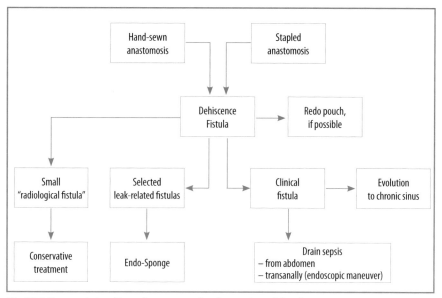

Fig 13.1 Proposed algorithm of treatment of early pouch-anal fistulas

cavity while draining the contaminated fluids. Based on the results, which require confirmation by prospective studies, Endo-Sponge could represent the treatment of choice in selected pouch anastomotic leak-related fistulas not requiring immediate surgery [28].

13.3.2 Late Fistulas

Late fistulas, occurring without initial anastomotic leak more than 6–12 months after ileostomy take-down, significantly impact the patient's quality of life, and present a technical challenge to the surgeon. This is particularly true in women in whom these fistulas usually take the form of a pouch-vaginal fistula, which is a source of considerable morbidity and has tremendous impact on the quality of life of the patient. The treatment of late fistulas is still controversial and, above all, is quite different in cases of pouch-anal as compared to pouch-vaginal tracts. The development of late perianal fistulas is not due to a septic phenomenon; therefore, this event must be considered not as a surgical complication, but rather as the deepening of an ulcer. In fact, the internal orifice of the fistula is almost always located below the anastomosis [29].

Moreover, although up to 5% of UC patients present with perianal disease, the discovery of a pouch-anal or pouch-vaginal fistula should be considered an alarming sign since it might represent a symptom of CD. The development of late pouch-anal or pouch-vaginal fistulas does not necessarily indicate CD; however, some authors believe that it is reasonable to classify patients with pouch-fistula as CD [30–32]. Fazio et al. [18] reported that more than 50% of patients with late perianal fistulas after IPAA suffer from CD. As highlighted above, this assumption is not necessarily true. There is no doubt, however, that the issue of the "evolutionary behavior" of indeterminate colitis has increased in the "pouch era", and this particular condition has become important since CD has widely been considered a contraindication to the fashioning of an ileoanal pouch.

The majority of the series reported in the literature show poor outcomes after IPAA in CD patients. Keighley [33] found a 52% rate of pouch failure in patients with CD. Mylonakis et al. [34], analyzing patients with CD who underwent IPAA and ileorenal anastomosis, reported a 47.8% rate of pouch excision as compared to an 8% rate of rectal excision. Similarly, Brown et al. [35] reported a 56% rate of pouch failure in CD patients as compared to 6% in UC patients and 10% in IC patients. On the other hand, Panis et al. [36] reported a 10% rate of pouch failure in highly selected patients with a confirmed preoperative diagnosis of CD. It should be pointed out that none of these patients had a past history of anal lesions or small bowel involvement. As a result of the data reported above, the therapeutic approach should be conservative, as for perianal fistulas in CD since the goal in these cases mainly consists in controlling the sepsis. It should be pointed out, however, that the introduction of anti-tumor necrosis factor (TNF)-alpha agents has changed this point of view, switching the ultimate treatment goal from controlling the sepsis to healing of fistulas.

The efficacy of older therapeutic agents, such as azathioprine (AZA)/ mercaptopurine (6-MP), and the newer TNF-antagonists infliximab (IFX) and adalimumab, in treating active luminal CD and maintaining remission has been well documented in non-pouch patients. In contrast, the current literature regarding the medical treatment of IPAA patients with CD-like complications is sparse. Even if a combined biosurgical approach could represent an effective resource, there is no general consensus regarding how to best medically manage this difficult-to-treat patient population.

13.3.2.1 Pouch-anal Fistulas

The aim of the current therapeutic approaches regarding the management of pouch-anal fistulas is to control sepsis in order to improve the patient's quality of life, limit the risk of pouch failure and possibly close and maintain closure of the fistula. Initial surgical treatment is mandatory for both simple and complex fistulas.

The main aspects to be taken into account when planning a strategy for the management of pouch-anal fistulas are to locate the origin of the fistula and its anatomy, evaluate the internal source of the fistulous tract (inflammation or stenosis) and sanitize the perineum with surgical control of local sepsis (abscess). Simple perianal fistulas may be treated with fistulotomy or seton placement.

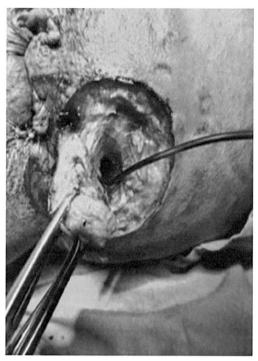

Fig. 13.2 Drainage of perianal sepsis: cone-like fistulectomy

For complex fistulas, treatment includes abscess drainage, a complete "cone-like" fistulectomy [37] and loose seton placement, the timing of removal depending on subsequent therapy. All patients should undergo surgical examination and sanitization of the perineum under anesthesia (EUA). Under general or spinal anesthesia, each fistula undergoes visual inspection, palpation and exploration with probes in order to identify all the fistulous tracts and abscesses. Purulent material is drained, and necrotic and inflamed tissues are excised. For each tract, a fistulectomy is performed, which consists of the excision of the tissue surrounding the fistula, starting from the skin adjacent to the external orifice and the subcutaneous fat tissue which encircles the entire tract, up to the source of the tract from the wall of the low rectum or the anal canal. The shape of the excision is conical ("cone-like technique") (Fig. 13.2), with a wide round base at the skin and the apex at the source of the fistula. This significantly reduces the risk of early closure of the external cutaneous surface and the subsequent risk of abscess recurrence. Finally, the seton, a non-absorbable suture monofilament, is inserted through each fistulous tract, using a probe, and left loosely inserted. This deep sanitization of the perineum limits the risk of worsening perianal sepsis with subsequent possible involvement of the sphincters by the septic process, and significantly improves the quality of life of patients. At the same time, it should be considered mandatory before initiating

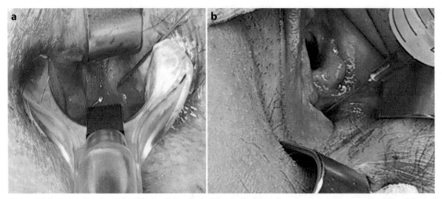

Fig 13.3 Local injection of infliximab into pouch-vaginal fistula: around the internal orifice (**a**) and along the fistulous tract (**b**)

any subsequent treatment, either medical or surgical, in order to ensure the best opportunity for success.

Medical therapy includes antibiotics and immunomodulators, mainly anti-TNF-alpha agents. In this respect, combined surgical and medical treatment with anti-TNF-alpha agents, as pointed out above, represents an attractive option, especially in patients with CD-related pouch-anal fistulas.

There have been several recent anecdotal reports of the successful use of TNF-antagonist therapy in treating this difficult-to-manage patient population [38–40], with encouraging results, even though the response in terms of real healing of the fistulous tracts is inferior to that reported in patients with complex Crohn's fistulas. In one case series of 17 patients with CD of the pouch, 47% had a complete symptom response and 23% had a partial response to a subcutaneous injection of adalimumab. Fistula response, however, was not as impressive since 60% of the patients showed no improvement at 4 weeks. The median follow-up in this series was short, only 8 weeks [38]. In a study by Viscido et al. [40], seven patients with refractory pouchitis complicated by fistulas were treated with a combination of IFX and AZA. Fistula closure was classified as complete, partial or none. At a median follow-up of 11 months, 57% of patients had a complete clinical response with complete closure of their fistulas.

A local injection of infliximab [37] can also be considered, especially in patients with contraindications for systemic use, despite the lack of controlled trials. The advantage of this therapeutic approach is that the biologic agent is injected into the mucosa surrounding the internal orifice representing the source of the fistula, allowing closure of the entire tract, avoiding false closure only at the external level which could lead to new abscess development. An anecdotal personal experience regarding 36 patients (11 with pouch-vaginal fistulas) (Fig. 13.3) showed a healing rate of 48% in pouch-anal and 9.1% in pouch-vaginal fistulas (data not published). This suggested that local injection is effective in patients with aggressive pouch-anal disease not treatable with surgery alone and not suitable for intravenous infliximab infusion due to the presence of contraindications.

A transanal mucosal advancement flap can be considered for patients with more complex fistulas after controlling any associated sepsis. This is substantially a variation on the mucosal advancement flap used for a high fistula-in-ano [41]. A cephalad-based U-shaped flap of mucosa and submucosa is mobilized from the ileal pouch; the internal opening is then excised and sutured at the internal muscle plane, and the flap is then advanced and sutured beyond the internal fistula opening. The advantages of this technique are that it is a quite straightforward procedure, it obliterates the septic focus and closes the internal opening, it does not impair the sphincters, it is repeatable, and it can be combined with overlapping sphincter reconstruction for anterior fistulas. Although the sphincter mechanism is not divided during the construction of an advancement flap, minor incontinence has been reported. Very few data regarding the results of this technique in pouch-anal fistulas have been reported in the literature. Ozuner et al. [32] showed a success rate of 45%; of the 24 patients who received advancement flaps, 10 had a successful outcome. In 14 patients, the initial ileal advancement flap failed. However, 5 patients had successful reoperations. In general, the success rate, even based on personal unpublished experience, is on the order of 50–60%, and there is no evidence that these results can be improved with a temporary diverting ileostomy [32]. Finally, it is important to stress that the procedure is contraindicated in the case of anastomotic stricture or perianastomotic inflammation. In these patients, the algorithm could be represented by the initial systemic or local administration of biologic drugs in order to obtain mucosal healing around the internal orifice, allowing subsequent surgical repair.

Mechanical systematic self-dilatation of the anastomosis with Hegars dilators and the topical administration of short-term steroids (enemas or suppositories) followed by sodium hyaluronate suppositories could be helpful in the mucosal healing process.

13.3.2.2 Pouch-vaginal Fistulas

Pouch-vaginal fistulas (PVF) are a source of considerable morbidity and significantly impact the quality of life of the patient. Only a few patients with PVF have few or no symptoms, with an occasional small amount of intestinal gas or minor discharge on the perineum. Unfortunately, the majority of patients present with more troublesome and embarrassing symptoms, such as vaginal discharge, variable amounts of fecal matter, gas discharge or recurrent vaginitis.

As indicated above, the development of a PVF represents a difficult problem and is an important factor leading to pouch failure. The incidence increases overtime after the ileal pouch has been fashioned and has been reported to range from 3–17% [14].

Wexner et al. [42] reported a pouch failure rate after PVF of 19% in a multicenter questionnaire sent to members of The American Society of Colon and Rectal Surgeons. A study from St. Mark's Hospital (London, UK) reported a pouch failure rate of 35% in patients who developed a PVF [43]. Another study reported a pouch failure rate of 22% in 60 patients at an average follow-up of 49 months [4].

Several predisposing factors are known to be associated with the development of a PVF, and these include technical factors, such as injury to the vagina or rectovaginal septum at the time of surgery [7, 8], septic factors, such as anastomotic leak leading to pelvic sepsis [4, 7] or, more frequently, disease-related factors such as late diagnosis of CD [4, 9]. The use of the double-stapled technique to construct the IPAA carries with it a risk of direct injury to the vagina at the time of surgery. This most likely results from the partial incorporation of the posterior vaginal wall within the circular staple line [7, 8]. There are conflicting reports as to whether the type of anastomosis (hand-sewn vs. stapled) during IPAA surgery predisposes to a PVF. A previous study by Lee et al. [44] found a substantially higher incidence of PVFs after a hand-sewn anastomosis as compared with the stapled technique. On the other hand, Groom et al. [5] found that the incidence of a PVF after a stapled anastomosis was twice that seen after a hand-sewn anastomosis. Two prospective randomized trials comparing hand-sewn and stapled IPAAs demonstrated no differences in the incidence of a PVF [6, 45].

Early onset of a PVF is likely to be associated with iatrogenic trauma to the rectovaginal septum during surgery or anastomotic complications whereas a late-onset PVF is correlated with the occurrence of cryptoglandular sepsis or the late diagnosis of CD [5, 42, 46, 47]. In fact, the internal orifice of a late PVF is almost always located below the anastomosis and, much less frequently, at the anastomosis or above it [14, 17, 48].

The position of the internal orifice related to the ileoanal anastomosis ("high" and "low") also influences the type of surgical approach. Transanal procedures are indicated for low fistulas while abdomino-perineal approach is appropriate for high fistulas. Furthermore, the treatment of choice for late pouch-vaginal fistulas is aggressive surgery since the non-surgical management or "minimal" surgical treatment results are disappointing and lead to poor functional outcome. This is the same behavior as in perianal CD (probably because it is perianal CD). Various surgical techniques have been used, and the majority of them have been adapted from techniques used to repair rectovaginal fistulas [49], even though with less success. The main transanal procedures are fistulectomy and seton placement, mucosal advancement flap (transanal or transvaginal), biological tissue plugs, ileal advancement flap, (Fazio), transposition of the gracilis muscle and direct suturing of the internal orifice. Abdominoperineal procedures include redo pouch and redo anastomosis, technically demanding procedures in which the long-term success rates do not exceed 50%.

The adverse effect on quality of life and the difficulty in managing the perineal discharge strongly suggest the fashioning of a diverting ileostomy, either before or at the same time as a repair. A stoma allows for resolution of the sepsis and inflammation even though there remains some concern [42, 44] as to whether defunctioning prior to the repair of a PVF is advantageous or not. A study found no significant differences in terms of final success between those patients who had been proximally diverted (29.7%) and those who had not (20.8%) [50]. Others have reported that an ileostomy seemed to have little impact on the chance of success, but the results could have been biased since it is only the worst cases which tend to be defunctioned [44].

Biologic plugs. The recent availability of collagen plugs for anal fistulas has led to the development of button plugs to treat a PVF. The technique involves suturing the button portion of the plug on the pouch side of the fistula with absorbable sutures. The button detaches within 4 weeks while the collagen matrix is left in situ. There are some reports of success with the button plug (success rates of approximately 55% at 16 weeks) [51] but such results were not maintained in the long term with 0 of 11 PVFs successfully healed at 2 years [52]. For this reason, the use of biological tissue plugs cannot be recommended for the management of a PVF.

Transanal pouch advancement flap. The results of this surgical repair technique, already described above, are slightly worse in terms of healing when compared to those for pouch-anal fistulas. In particular, Shah et al. [46] reported a success rate of 44% with an advancement flap procedure done perianally. Twenty-two out of 44 patients who underwent this procedure had a recurrence. Lee et al. [44] had a slightly higher success rate (50%, 10/20 patients). Additional analysis showed a marginal difference in the healing rate between patients with ileostomy and those proceeding directly to repair. In another recent study [4], the successful healing rate of a PVF using an advancement flap was 42% after primary repair and 66% when performed secondarily after a different procedure.

Transanal pouch advancement/revision. A technique of transanal disconnection of the ileal pouch from the IPAA, transanal advancement of the pouch and resuturing at the dentate line has been described for patients with significant stricturing at the IPAA. This technique can be employed in patients with a PVF, especially in slender patients with a safe mobility of the pouch, above the anastomosis. The advantage of this technique is that it transposes healthy, full thickness tissue to the region of the fistula in a full thickness manner [41]. Heriot et al. [43] showed that the procedure was successful in one out of two patients.

Tissue interposition: graciloplasty. The fundamental aim of using tissue flaps is to place healthy tissue between the two fistulous openings. A variety of techniques to transpose healthy muscle between the rectum and the vagina for the repair of rectovaginal fistulas have been described. Only the gracilis muscle flap has been used for the repair of a PVF. The gracilis can be detached from its

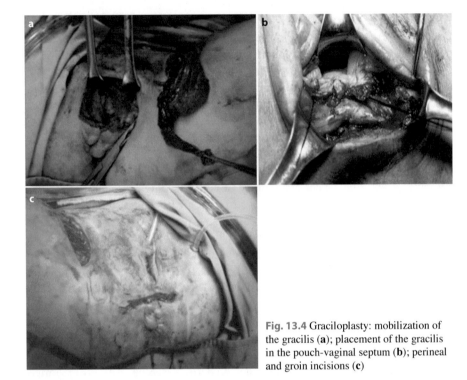

Fig. 13.4 Graciloplasty: mobilization of the gracilis (**a**); placement of the gracilis in the pouch-vaginal septum (**b**); perineal and groin incisions (**c**)

insertion, mobilized, tunneled subcutaneously, and secured between the pouch and the vagina. This provides a well-nourished, vascularized piece of tissue with the slight disadvantage of the small extra incisions required to mobilize the gracilis muscle (Fig. 13.4) [53]. There are three series which report the outcomes of a gracilis interposition flap for a PVF. In 2008, Wexner et al. [54] first described their experience regarding the use of the gracilis interposition flap for the treatment of a PVF. The procedure was successful in 1 out of the 2 patients who underwent the procedure. The patient in whom the flap repair failed had undergone multiple previous repairs for a PVF and was diagnosed with CD. The average success rate is approximately 80% [17, 53, 54]. In general, interposition flaps are particularly useful after previous failed repairs as well as when abdominal procedures are contraindicated. The majority of series show a high morbidity of approximately 33–50%, including perineal wound infection, urethral stricture, fever, urinary retention and perineal bleeding [17].

Tissue interposition transabdominal approach. A PVF which arises from the midbody of the ileal pouch requires a transabdominal approach. This carries a significant risk of loss of the pouch [46, 55]. At laparotomy, the pouch is mobilized down to the pelvic floor with careful dissection between the vagina and the anterior wall of the ileal pouch to avoid unintentional damage to the anterior wall of the pouch. While it is sometimes possible to identify, disconnect and repair the fistula, and carry out an omentoplasty, it is more commonly necessary to transect at the anal outlet, excise the pouch outlet, curette and close the track and then carry out a hand-sewn pouch-anal anastomosis. It is then appropriate to cover the new anastomosis with an ileostomy. Such procedures are technically demanding and probably best left in the hands of surgeons and institutions with a high-volume pouch practice. A review of the literature reveals a 40–50% risk of postoperative morbidity with abdominal procedures, albeit with success rates of 50–60% [55].

Local versus abdominal procedures. Four studies [16, 46, 48, 56] included both local and abdominal procedures. None were randomized controlled trials, and none included direct comparison. Tsujinaka et al. [48] showed that the successful management of a PVF situated at or below the anastomosis was achieved with local procedures, including transanal ileal advancement in 73% of patients. Transabdominal procedures were successful for a PVF above the anastomosis in 67% of cases. They concluded that abdominal procedures should be performed for high fistulas and local procedures for low fistulas. Zinicola et al. [56] from St. Mark's (London) also confirmed that the success rates were high when the abdominal approach was employed for high fistulas. Nine out of 11 patients treated with an abdominal procedure had successful repairs, although two patients needed repeat procedures to achieve success.

13.4   Conclusions

Fistulization from the ileal reservoir to various sites may be a distressing complication of pouch surgery which can lead to loss of the pouch. No single factor was identified as a cause of pouch fistulas. Once fistulas develop, various salvage procedures can safely be attempted in a successful fashion and will restore pouch function in approximately 50–60% of the patients. Combined biosurgical treatment shows preliminary encouraging results and should be considered as the first line strategy. Of the surgical procedures proposed, none seems to be superior to the others, and there are no randomized studies to our knowledge. The choice of procedure should be based on the clinical features and history of the patient and the fistula. Thus, the surgeon should be prepared to use different approaches or techniques to achieve optimum success.

References

1.   Hahnloser D, Pemberton JH, Wolff BG et al (2007) Results at up to 20 years after ileal pouch-anal anastomosis for chronic ulcerative colitis. Br J Surg 94(3):333–340

2. Tekkis PP, Fazio VW, Remzi F et al (2005) Risk factors associated with ileal pouch-related fistula following restorative proctocolectomy. Br J Surg 92(10):1270–1276
3. Gorgun E, Remzi FH (2004) Complications of ileoanal pouches. Clin Colon Rectal Surg 17(1):43–55
4. Mallick IH, Hull TL, Remzi FH et al (2014) Management and outcome of pouch-vaginal fistulas after IPAA surgery. Dis Colon Rectum 57(4):490–496
5. Groom JS, Nicholls RJ, Hawley PR, Phillips RK (1993) Pouch-vaginal fistula. Br J Surg 80(7):936–940
6. Luukkonen P, Järvinen H (1993) Stapled vs hand-sutured ileoanal anastomosis in restorative proctocolectomy. A prospective, randomized study. Arch Surg 128(4):437–440
7. Braveman JM, Schoetz DJ Jr, Marcello PW et al (2004) The fate of the ileal pouch in patients developing Crohn's disease. Dis Colon Rectum 47(10):1613–1619
8. Melton GB, Fazio VW, Kiran RP et al (2008) Long-term outcomes with ileal pouch-anal anastomosis and Crohn's disease: pouch retention and implications of delayed diagnosis. Ann Surg 248(4):608–616
9. Tulchinsky H, Hawley PR, Nicholls J (2003) Long-term failure after restorative procto-colectomy for ulcerative colitis. Ann Surg 238(2):229–234
10. Sagar PM, Dozois RR, Wolff BG (1996) Long-term results of ileal pouch-anal anastomosis in patients with Crohn's disease. Dis Colon Rectum 39(8):893–898
11. Pellino G, Sciaudone G, Miele E et al (2014) Functional outcomes and quality of life after restorative proctocolectomy in paediatric patients: a case-control study. Gastroenterol Res Pract 2014:340341
12. Schwartz DA, Herdman CR (2004) Review article: The medical treatment of Crohn's perianal fistulas. Aliment Pharmacol Ther 19(9):953–967
13. Felley C, Mottet C, Juillerat P et al (2005) Fistulizing Crohn's disease. Digestion 71(1):26–28
14. Lolohea S, Lynch AC, Robertson GB, Frizelle FA (2005) Ileal pouch-anal anastomosis-vaginal fistula: a review. Dis Colon Rectum 48(9):1802–1810
15. Paye F, Penna C, Chiche L et al (1996) Pouch-related fistula following restorative proctocolectomy. Br J Surg 83(11):1574–1577
16. Johnson PM, O'Connor BI, Cohen Z, McLeod RS (2005) Pouch-vaginal fistula after ileal pouch-anal anastomosis: treatment and outcomes. Dis Colon Rectum 48(6):1249–1253
17. Maslekar S, Sagar PM, Harji D et al (2012) The challenge of pouch-vaginal fistulas: a systematic review. Tech Coloproctol 16(6):405–414
18. Fazio VW, Tekkis PP, Remzi F et al (2003) Quantification of risk for pouch failure after ileal pouch anal anastomosis surgery. Ann Surg 238(4):605–614; discussion 614–617
19. Nisar PJ, Kiran RP, Shen B et al (2011) Factors associated with ileoanal pouch failure in patients developing early or late pouch-related fistula. Dis Colon Rectum 54(4):446–453
20. Bell SJ, Halligan S, Windsor AC et al (2003) Response of fistulating Crohn's disease to infliximab treatment assessed by magnetic resonance imaging. Aliment Pharmacol Ther 17(3):387–393
21. Schwartz DA, Wiersema MJ, Dudiak KM et al (2001) A comparison of endoscopic ultrasound, magnetic resonance imaging, and exam under anesthesia for evaluation of Crohn's perianal fistulas. Gastroenterology 121(5):1064–1072
22. Kariv R, Plesec T, Remzi et al (2007) Pyloric gland metaplasia – a novel histological marker for refractory pouchitis and Crohn's disease of the pouch. Gastroenterology 132(Suppl 2):A132
23. Rasul I, Wilson SR, MacRae H et al (2004) Clinical and radiological responses after infliximab treatment for perianal fistulizing Crohn's disease. Am J Gastroenterol 99(1):82–88
24. Whitlow CB, Opelka FG, Gathright JB Jr, Beck DE (1997) Treatment of colorectal and ileoanal anastomotic sinuses. Dis Colon Rectum 40(7):760–763
25. McGuire BB, Brannigan AE, O'Connel PR (2007) Ileal pouch-anal anastomosis. Br J Surg 94(7):812–823

26. Poggioli G, Marchetti F, Selleri S et al (1993) Redo pouches: salvaging of failed ileal pouch-anal anastomoses. Dis Colon Rectum 36(5):492–496
27. Gardenbroek TJ, Musters GD, Buskens CJ et al (2015) Early reconstruction of the leaking ileal pouch-anal anastomosis: a novel solution to an old problem. Colorectal Dis 17(5):426–432
28. Rottoli M, Di Simone MP, Vallicelli C et al (2018) Endoluminal vacuum-assisted therapy as treatment for anastomotic leak after ileal pouch-anal anastomosis: a pilot study. Tech Coloproctol 22(3):223–229
29. Parks AG, Nicholls RJ (1978) Proctocolectomy without ileostomy for ulcerative colitis. Br Med J 2(6130):85–88
30. Marcello PW, Schoetz DJ Jr, Roberts PL et al (1997) Evolutionary changes in the pathologic diagnosis after the ileoanal pouch procedure. Dis Colon Rectum 40(3):263–269
31. Colombel JF, Ricart E, Loftus EV Jr et al (2003) Management of Crohn's disease of the ileo-anal pouch with infliximab. Am J Gastroenterol 98(10):2239–2244
32. Ozuner G, Hull T, Lee P, Fazio VW (1997) What happens to a pelvic pouch when a fistula develops? Dis Colon Rectum 40(5):543–547
33. Keighley MR (2000) The final diagnosis in pouch patients for presumed ulcerative colitis may change to Crohn's Disease: patients should be warned of the consequences. Acta Chir Iugosl 47(4 Suppl 1):27–31
34. Mylonakis E, Allan RN, Keighley MR (2001) How does pouch construction for a final diagnosis of Crohn's disease compare with ileoproctostomy for established Crohn's proctocolitis? Dis Colon Rectum 44(8):1137–1142; discussion 1142–1143
35. Brown CJ, MacLean AR, Cohen Z et al (2005) Crohn's disease and indeterminate colitis and the ileal pouch-anal anastomosis: outcomes and patterns of failure. Dis Colon Rectum 48(8):1542–1549
36. Panis Y, Poupard B, Nemeth J et al (1996) Ileal pouch/anal anastomosis for Crohn's disease. Lancet 347(9005):854–857
37. Poggioli G, Laureti S, Pierangeli F et al (2005) Local injection of infliximab for the treatment of perianal Crohn's disease. Dis Colon Rectum 48(4):768–774
38. Ferrante M, D'Haens G, Dewit O et al; Belgian IBD Research Group (2010) Efficacy of infliximab in refractory pouchitis and Crohn's disease-related complications of the pouch: a Belgian case series. Inflamm Bowel Dis 16(2):243–249
39. Viscido A, Habib FI, Kohn A et al (2003) Infliximab in refractory pouchitis complicated by fistulae following ileo-anal pouch for ulcerative colitis. Aliment Pharmacol Ther 17(10):1263–1271
40. Ricart E, Panaccione R, Loftus EV et al (1999) Successful management of Crohn's disease of the ileoanal pouch with infliximab. Gastroenterology 117(2):429–432
41. Fazio VW, Tjandra JJ (1992) Pouch advancement and neoileoanal anastomosis for anastomotic stricture and anovaginal fistula complicating restorative proctocolecotmy. Br J Surg 79(7):694–696
42. Wexner SD, Rothenberger DA, Jensen L et al (1989) Ileal pouch vaginal fistulas: incidence, etiology, and management. Dis Colon Rectum 32(6):460–465
43. Heriot AG, Tekkis PP, Smith JJ et al (2005) Management and outcome of pouch-vaginal fistulas following restorative proctocolectomy. Dis Colon Rectum 48(3):451–458
44. Lee PY, Fazio VW, Church JM et al (1997) Vaginal fistula following restorative proctocolectomy. Dis Colon Rectum 40(7):752–759
45. Choen S, Tsunoda A, Nicholls RJ (1991) Prospective randomized trial comparing anal function after hand sewn ileoanal anastomosis with mucosectomy versus stapled ileoanal anastomosis without mucosectomy in restorative proctocolectomy. Br J Surg 78(4):430–434
46. Shah NS, Remzi F, Massmann A et al (2003) Management and treatment outcome of pouch-vaginal fistulas following restorative proctocolectomy. Dis Colon Rectum 46(7):911–917
47. Burke D, van Laarhoven CJ, Herbst F, Nicholls RJ (2001) Transvaginal repair of pouch-vaginal fistula. Br J Surg 88(2):241–245

48. Tsujinaka S, Ruiz D, Wexner SD et al (2006) Surgical management of pouch-vaginal fistula after restorative proctocolectomy. J Am Coll Surg 202(6):912–918
49. Mazier WP, Senagore AJ, Schiesel EC (1995) Operative repair of anovaginal and rectovaginal fistulas. Dis Colon Rectum 38(1):4–6
50. Gorfine SR, Fichera A, Harris MT, Bauer JJ (2003) Long-term results of salvage surgery for septic complications after restorative proctocolectomy: does fecal diversion improve outcome? Dis Colon Rectum 46(10):1339–1344
51. Gonsalves S, Sagar P, Lengyel J et al (2009) Assessment of the efficacy of the rectovaginal button fistula plug for the treatment of ileal pouch-vaginal and rectovaginal fistulas. Dis Colon Rectum 52(11):1877–1881
52. Gajsek U, McArthur DR, Sagar PM (2011) Long-term efficacy of the button fistula plug in the treatment of ileal pouch-vaginal and Crohn's-related rectovaginal fistulas. Dis Colon Rectum 54(8):999–1002
53. Zmora O, Potenti FM, Wexner SD et al (2003) Gracilis muscle transposition for iatrogenic rectourethral fistula. Ann Surg 237(4):483–487
54. Wexner SD, Ruiz DE, Genua J et al (2008) Gracilis muscle interposition for the treatment of rectourethral, rectovaginal, and pouch-vaginal fistulas: results in 53 patients. Ann Surg 248(1):39–43
55. MacLean AR, O'Connor B, Parkes R et al (2002) Reconstructive surgery for failed ileal pouch-anal anastomosis: a viable surgical option with acceptable results. Dis Colon Rectum 45(7):880–886
56. Zinicola R, Wilkinson KH, Nicholls RJ (2003) Ileal pouch-vaginal fistula treated by abdominoanal advancement of the ileal pouch. Br J Surg 90(11):1434–1435

Printed in the United States
By Bookmasters